|| श्रीं ||

Kālāmṛta 2013

Immortal Vedic Wisdom for Every Day Life

Kālāmṛta 2013

All astrological data was compiled by

Puṇḍit Mahesh Shastri of

www.mypanchang.com

Printed in the United States

ISBN 978-1-4675-3361-4

Email: kalamrita@gmail.com

Website: www.kalamrita.com

We humbly dedicate Kālāmṛta
to our Sadguru - Śrī Mātā Amṛtānandamayī
&
to the living embodiment of
Dhanvantari's grace - Vaidya Shreerang Galgali.

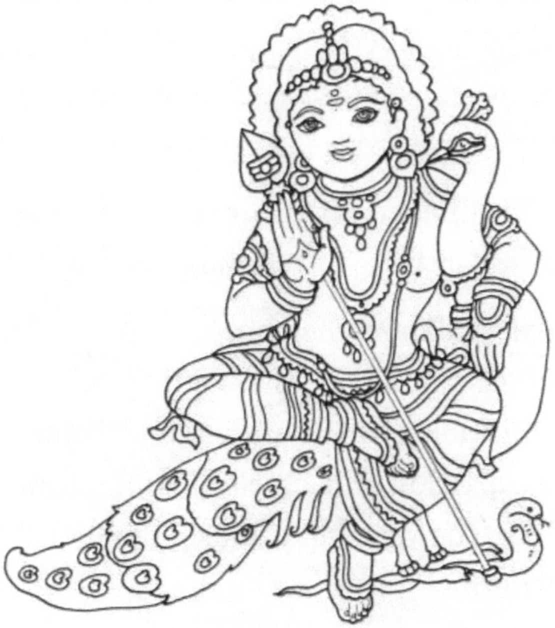

ॐ लोकाः समस्ताः सुखिनो भवन्तू

Kālāmṛta is a mapping of time using the sidereal zodiac or Nirayaṇa Cakra, as it is known in India. Those familiar with Western astrological calendars will find recognizable elements here, including the phases of the Moon, the daily sign of the Moon and many other features of an almanac. Also included are articles on Hasta Sāmudrika Śāstra (Palmistry) as well as articles on Vedic astrology, including an article on eclipses.

Kālāmṛta is divided into four sections based on the seasons. Both Vedic and Western holidays are listed.

Each year, Kālāmṛta celebrates a deity. This year, we honor Lord Dakṣiṇāmūrti. Although you might not be familiar with this deity, we invite you meet him through the many pictures, articles and stories illuminating the sacred principles behind the worship of Dakṣiṇāmūrti, Adi-guru, the teacher of teachers.

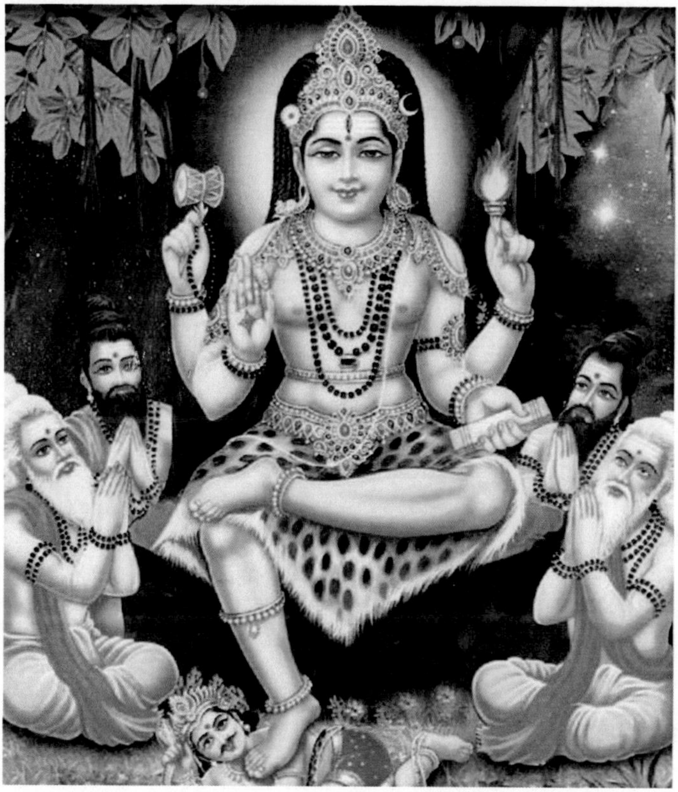

Kālāmṛta 2013 Table of Contents

Dedicated to
Śrī Mātā Amṛtānandamayī Devī

Through her extraordinary acts of love and self-sacrifice, Mātā Amṛtānandamayī or Amma (Mother) as she is affectionately known, has endeared herself to millions of people around the world. Offering a spiritual blessing to everyone who comes to her in the form of a hug, She holds them close to her heart in a loving embrace. Amma shares her boundless love with all - regardless of their beliefs, who they are or why they have come to her. In this simple yet powerful way, Amma is transforming the lives of countless people and helping their hearts to blossom, one embrace at a time. In the past 30 years, Amma has physically hugged more than 24 million people from all parts of the world. Her tireless spirit of dedication to uplifting others has inspired a vast network of charitable activities through which people are discovering the beauty and sense of peace that come from selflessly serving others. Amma teaches that the Divine exists in everything, sentient and insentient. Perceiving this underlying unity in all things is not only the essence of spirituality but also the means to end all suffering. Amma's teachings are universal. Whenever she is asked about her religion, she replies that her religion is Love. She does not ask anyone to believe in God or to change their faith but only to inquire into their own real nature, and to believe in themselves. For more information on Amma and her activities, please visit her website: www.amma.org

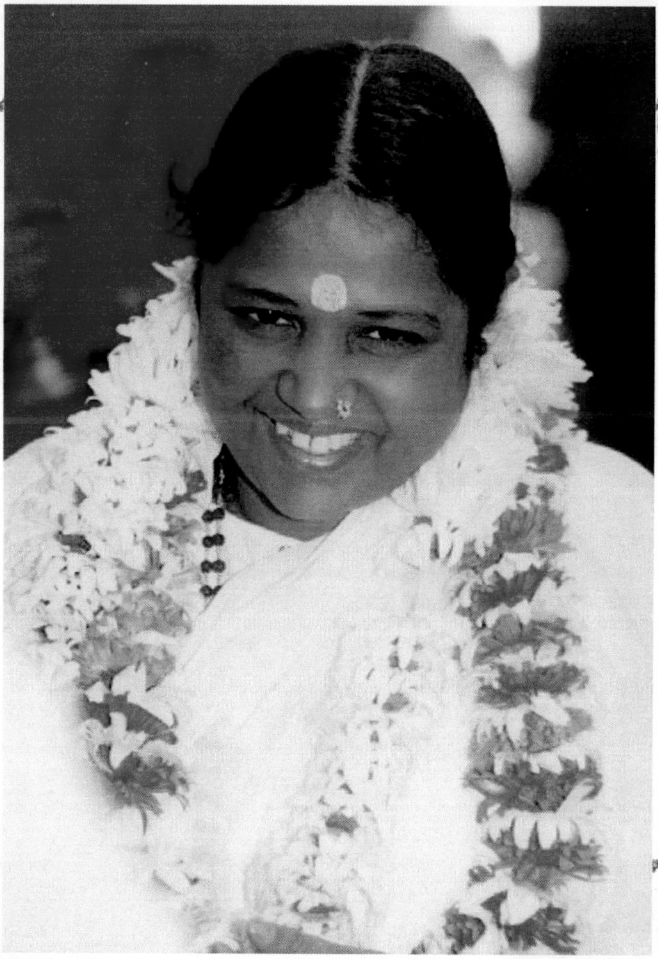

ॐ

Welcome

In 1726 a certain young man only in his mid-twenties proposed thirteen virtues, which he found to be essential to the well lived life. He pledged that he would live by these virtues daily. This enthusiastic list of morals shaped the young man into a leader of an emerging nation. He was none other than Mr. Benjamin Franklin. In his autobiography, Franklin instructs the reader on how to integrate his thirteen virtues into their lives. He said that it is better to practice one virtue at a time, rather than working with all of them at once, otherwise, we run the risk of becoming overwhelmed.

In this spirit, we present one of Ben's picks for the greatest of all virtues; Industry. He defines it as such: "[Concerning] industry. Lose no time; be always employ'd in something useful; cut off all unnecessary actions." He later warns that without employing industry, "Lost time is never found." Even before those magnanimous lines were penned by Franklin, people throughout the ages have suffered the regret of having 'wasted time'; whether it is an afternoon lost to laziness or an ill spent stage of life, all of humanity has tasted the bitter drink of lost time.

The beauty of the virtue of Industry lies in its timelessness. Whether it is Franklin's era or our own, industriousness is of supreme value. A true virtue also has the ability to transcend culture and the virtue of industry does so effortlessly – found in the Vedic tradition it could be translated as 'Karma' which means 'action'. Karma is so highly esteemed that it has been validated as a legitimate path to God-Realization, called 'Karma Yoga'. This approach to industry is not oriented toward being a busy bee, as might be understood by Ben's definition but instead stresses the importance of being in right relationship with all of our actions. Karma yoga, like Mr. Franklin, encourages us to be usefully engaged and to strive to eliminate 'unnecessary actions'. The difference between karma yoga and Ben's wholehearted exploration of *industry* is this: while Ben spent a lifetime trying to codify and define what true industry really is, the tradition of karma yoga has been firmly established for countless ages, no tinkering required.

The trifold idea of not losing time, always being engaged in something useful and cutting off all unnecessary action is alive and well in the principles of karma yoga. Yet karma yoga is far more elegant than just encouraging us to not waste time and to get busy! Karma yoga encourages us to engage in our daily duties, whatever they may be; the distinction between karma yoga and 'industry' lies in the mindset we cultivate while going about our work. The mindset of karma yoga is one of trusting in the Lord so completely that we accept what may come as a result of whatever we do as his blessing bestowed upon us. By fostering this attitude, no time is ever wasted, since we are constantly engaged in the beautiful dance between our actions and the Lord's blessing being showered upon us. It is only when we lose that attitude that we begin to regret how we have spent our time. When we act from our heart and trust that the Universe will give us exactly what we need, then no time is ever wasted. We are always learning, growing and deepening our relationship with God and ourselves. So rather than despairing about our lost promotion or bread that didn't rise, we actually can have a different perspective, one that allows us to not get what we expected and still be absolutely okay with that because we trust that God is always giving us exactly what we need, when we need it.

In that spirit, we welcome you to Kālāmṛta 2013. We are happy

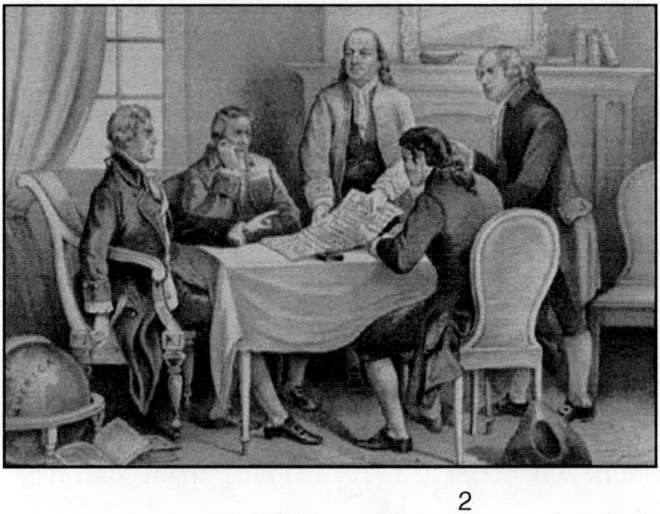

to present to you a wonderful edition this year. In addition to daily astrological listings, Kālāmṛta offers articles on Vedic astrology, including a fascinating article about eclipses. Also, this year we feature articles on Hasta Sāmudrika, otherwise known as Vedic Palmistry.

Many different scholars and practitioners have joined together to create Kālāmṛta. The product of this collaborative effort serves as a gateway to further our understanding of the sacred and powerful tradition of ancient India. Included are several articles illustrating the use of this almanac so even a beginner can successfully navigate the tables that we have provided with ease and delight. The Vedic and Western holidays presented are accurately determined and can be used by those wishing to commence their celebrations at the correct time.

Each year, Kālāmṛta celebrates a deity. This year, we celebrate Lord Dakṣiṇāmūrti. Inside, you'll find articles on Dakṣiṇāmūrti, who he is, his place in the Vedic Sampradāya, various līlā stories about his sportings and articles helping to properly understand his iconography. We offer this almanac to lovers of the Vedic tradition and its auxiliary branches and to those who are just becoming familiarized with the tradition as well. Please join us and the growing numbers of others like yourself who follow Vedic holidays, love yoga and those who are interested in Vedic Astrology, will all benefit from the use of this almanac.

May divine grace be ever upon us all. May lord Dakṣiṇāmūrti bless us. May we continue to become increasingly aware of the blessing that is *time*. Welcome to the wonderful world of Kālāmṛta!

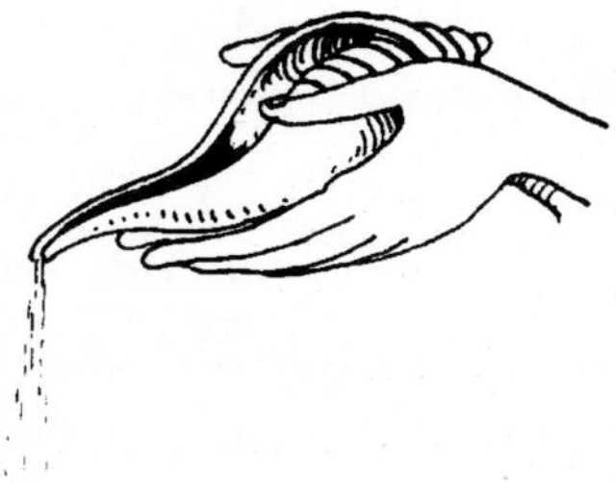

Introduction

We want you to love Kālāmṛta . It is our passion and we are dedicated to sharing it with you. Kālāmṛta is not *just* a day planner used to jot down appointments and reminders in. There is something infinitely more grand going on within these pages. We want you to understand the magic of time. Just in the same way that you have become more aware of your body and breath through Yoga, more aware of your mental constructs through meditation now you can bring the awareness of *time* into your daily life through the use of Kālāmṛta. Certainly, Kālāmṛta can be used as an appointment keeper – but we think it is far more enchanting to delve in deeper, to bring the awareness of time into your daily life. Kālāmṛta is a life-style; it is a community of people dedicated to living life more fully, more successfully. Welcome home!

We have packed each and every page with the tools you need to befriend the most powerful energy there is – TIME. The greatest temples, leaders and even ideas, will one day crumple under this merciless force . Time truly can be our foe or our most precious ally. When we resist the flow of time, we fight a force that cannot be beat. We will age, our precious belongs will eventually wear out and perhaps most cruelly of all – nothing will ever stay the same. Everything is under the spell of time and therefore, our children grow, our lovers age and our knees aren't as forgiving as they once were. Fight it – but time still marches on

Almost all spiritual traditions invite us to take a different perspective – befriend time. Let it be your teacher. Let it lead you through the dance of life. By accepting the relentless and unstoppable movement of time, we can relax into the ever changing world that we are constantly swimming in. Accepting that nothing in the world will remain constant, we can begin to develop fortitude. Fortitude cultivated with awareness is called titikṣā. This can be translated as 'accommodation' or the ability to accept the circumstances that life presents. Titīkṣā allows all things to be as they are without the need to change them. Time is always teaching us that no matter how hard we try, even the most wonderful experience will not last. Since nothing in the world is eternal, does that mean we should just stand aside and allow things to happen with no self - effort? Not at all. The tradition accounts for a certain amount of free will and therefore gives us tools to co-participate with our world. Included in that ever-handy tool kit is the knowledge of how to begin to flow in time in a harmonious and optimal way. For truly, mastering time sets us free.

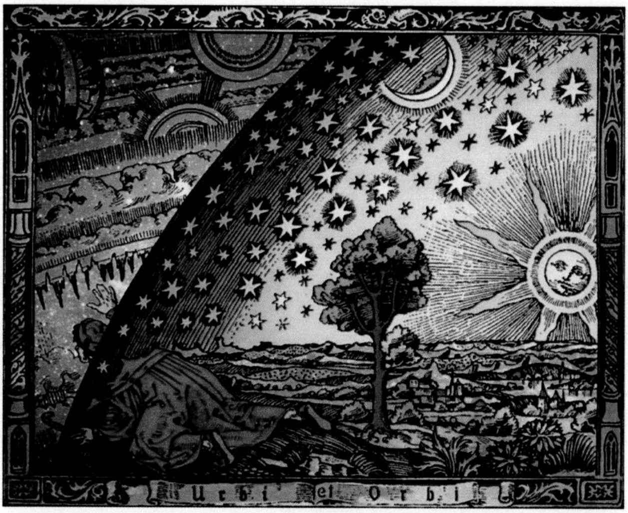

This begins with the awareness that one of the most powerful expressions of free will is in the intentional use of time. Learning a few basic principles about the inner workings of time and about the calendar and using this knowledge to initiate activities at proper times liberates us from the drudgery of not being 'in the flow'. Another component to mastering time is to lift the veil that permeates our world to see that though everything that comes into existence is time bound. There is only one thing which is not bound by time - Ātmā. Ātmā is the supreme consciousness that permeates everything, including each and every one of us. So even though time appears to decimate everything in its path, it can never touch our true nature, through it all, our true essence remains untouched.

Kālāmṛta is dedicated to pursing the mastery of not only time but of our very own Self. Thanks for joining us – we're glad you're here!

An Introduction to Dakṣiṇāmūrti

This year, Kālāmṛta honors and celebrates the potent wisdom of Lord Dakṣiṇāmūrti. Here, we will take a closer look at the being of Dakṣiṇāmūrti so as to better understand the deep potency of his teaching.

An incarnation of Lord Śiva, Dakṣiṇāmūrti is recognized as the first amongst teachers; the guru of the gurus, a supreme manifestation of the Divine. *Dakṣiṇā* in Sanskrit means South and *Mūrti* can be translated as form, so Dakṣiṇāmūrti is an embodiment of God who is seated facing the South. Bedecked in a rich tapestry of symbolism, Dakṣiṇāmūrti's very form, when meditated upon, transmits knowledge of the supporting agent of all other subjects – Ātmā Jñāna or Self Knowledge. In this article, we take a step into deeper understanding of the symbolism surrounding Dakṣiṇāmūrti and the accoutrements to his silent exposition of the Self.

Whereas most deities are depicted facing North or East, Dakṣiṇāmūrti faces South. From an astrological perspective, the Southern direction symbolizes death and completions, the ending of cycles

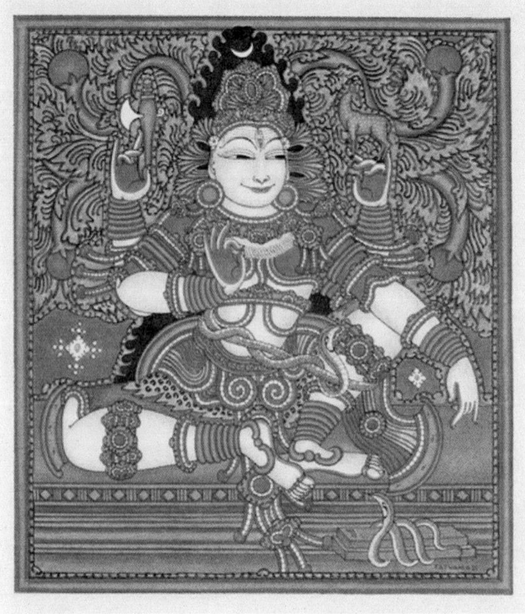

which make way for the beginning of new ones. One should not be alarmed that Śrī Dakṣiṇāmūrti is seated faced death; in fact, he faces South to illustrate that it is a perfect master who has conquered the cycles of birth and death through their knowledge of the Self. As the Southern direction is equated with death, the North is conversely associated with life. In pure compassion

Dakṣiṇāmūrti sits facing South, thus permitting his students to realize the goal of life and attain that knowledge that flows from the North: the knowledge of the Absolute and of the relationship between the individual Soul and its part-and-parcel being-ness with the Universal Soul. As he has already attained the mastery of the Self, Dakṣiṇāmūrti need not worry about the direction in which he faces during meditation – he has gone beyond the limitation of both space and time as well as the directions. This part of the iconography is instructive to us, for when sitting in meditation we too can practice facing North, in the direction that symbolizes life and knowledge.

In his right hand, Dakṣiṇāmūrti makes the divine gesture known as the *Cin-Mudra*, literally, "Gesture of Consciousness". The Cin-Mudra is made by folding the index finger over halfway, its tip held under the curled thumb, while the rest hand is held upright with the middle, ring and little fingers pointing up. Cin-mudra symbolizes the ego that has completely submitted to the higher Consciousness and has deep yogic implications. The energy currents within the body connect the individual ego with the index finger. Similarly, the thumb represents the Supreme Reality – that which exists independently of the rest of the hand, yet without which the hand is so woefully incomplete. The middle finger that is held erect is connected through the subtle channels to the bodily senses – sight, touch, taste, hearing and smell. From the ring finger runs a subtle current to the mind. Finally, the little finger branches out to the entire rest of the physical body. Therefore, by restraining the egoic index finger firmly with the thumb of the Supreme Reality, Dakṣiṇāmūrti shows spiritual seekers that the way to God consciousness lies in a constant remembrance that the ego is nothing compared to the vastness that is God. In the *Śiva Bhakta Vilāsam*, Śiva says, "May you be fully enlightened by this Cin-Mudra of mine and

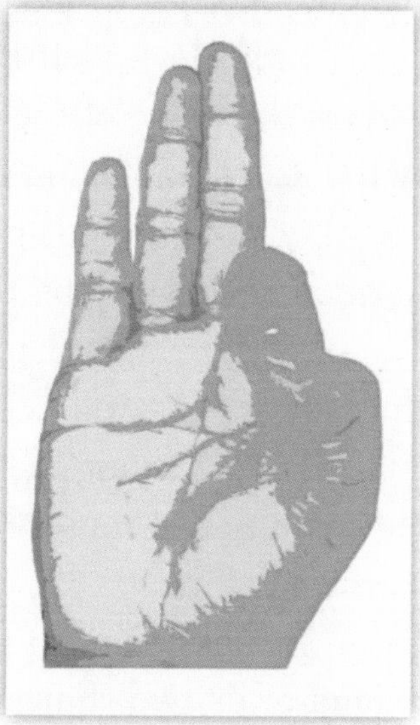

escape the vicious cycle of birth and death." Just as the middle, ring and little fingers are held aloft once the index finger has submitted to the thumb; the senses, mind and body will still operate and function but with the newfound freedom of remembrance of the Self. Once the ego is resigned to the Self, the senses, mind and body all flow upward with a sustained surge of divine intention for the good of all of creation – rather than feeding the lower nature of acting because of likes and dislikes.

In his upper right hand, Dakṣiṇāmūrti holds a rosary made of rudrākṣa seeds, which He uses to continuously chant a mantra or divine prayer. This imagery is used to remind us that Dakṣiṇāmūrti is ever immersed in a mood of remembering the Self of All, through deep and unbroken reflection.

In his lower left hand, Dakṣiṇāmūrti holds the holy Veda. The Veda is the name of the canonical spiritual text "seen" and cognized by the Ṛṣis in millennia past, the Veda was then codified into written text. Divided into four parts, the Vedas were "seen" from the highest spiritual realms by the blemishless sages that lived in ancient India. Cognized thus from a place of ultimate purity, the Vedas are both eternally true as well as eternally applicable even to us as modern day humans. By holding the holy Veda, Dakṣiṇāmūrti urges our constant remembrance of those things in life that are pure and good for all of human-kind.

In Dakṣiṇāmūrti's upper left hand is a pot of fire. This can remind of us two things - the first is the exhortation to "live in the world but not of it." The fire in the pot represents the worldly lifestyle wherein one normally does not take the time to remember the Lord. These temporary and transitory entrapments we should resist. The pot of flames held aloft by Dakṣiṇāmūrti also reminds of the need to kindle and nourish the spiritual fire within us. Consciousness or *caitanya* flows upwards like a flame when directed in a spiritual way whereas that same caitanya flows down like water when our focus is on mundane senses and their objects of experiences.

Dakṣiṇāmūrti is seated under the *vaṭa* tree. Botanically known as *ficus indica*, commonly known as the banyan tree and Āyurvedically known as a kalpavṛkṣa or "wish fulfilling tree," the vaṭa tree is considered to be a very important tree because all parts of the tree are beneficial to one's health. Both the edible fruits, tender leaves, bark and new shoots all have various healing properties. This includes – to name a few - increasing male potency, healing gynecological disorders, and as a digestive aid. Dakṣiṇāmūrti, the disseminator of Absolute Knowledge which gives his devotees life in the truest sense, is akin to this wish-fulfilling and life-giving tree. When a vaṭa tree grows, its branches produce vines that dangle and grow towards the ground. When these vines reach the ground, new roots shoot out at the earth causing what was once a vine to now become a new supporting trunk for the original branch. In this way, the long armed branches of the vaṭa tree can grow to be hundreds of feet long, yet barely hovering six feet over the ground with its trellis of supporting pseudo trunks. This makes an ideal canopy for Dakṣiṇāmūrti to sit under whether meditating or revealing Supreme Knowledge to his students. Protected from both the *krūra* noon-day Sun as well as the downpour of the Indian monsoon, Dakṣiṇāmūrti sits in harmony with nature in unbroken contemplation on the Absolute.

At the feet of Dakṣiṇāmūrti are a group of sages, well-advanced in years. One might wonder at the incongruity of the youthful form of Dakṣiṇāmūrti instructing a group of aged sages who sit in rapt attention at his feet. Dakṣiṇāmūrti is depicted as a youth because holding the knowledge of the Supreme Reality in his mind creates such vibrancy in Dakṣiṇāmūrti that his external form has no choice but to conform to his internal mood and remain ever-youthful. The inner Self is eternal, unchanging and spotlessly pure. Holding such a poignant remembrance in his mind allows its perennial vibrations to wash over Dakṣiṇāmūrti, keeping him free of even the slightest hint of decrepitude.

Dakṣiṇāmūrti's resplendent foot rests upon a demon that is known by the name Apasmāra. This name can be literally translated as confusion, want of memory or forgetfulness. Like an unbroken stream of oil being poured from one container to another, Dakṣiṇāmūrti banishes forgetfulness of the Self and immerses himself in its flow of purifying waters.

If one looks keenly, they will notice that Dakṣiṇāmūrti has different earrings in his two ears. In his right ear is a male earring and in his left ear is a female earring. Dakṣiṇāmūrti is also a manifestation of Ardhanārīśvara, the dual male/female form of Lord Siva. With these adornments, Dakṣiṇāmūrti shows the devotee that after one has realized the Absolute, the distinction between "I and mine", attachment and aversion, and perhaps the deepest association that the incarnated soul can have, identification with being male or female, is transcended.

Dakṣiṇāmūrti is the living and breathing embodiment of the knowledge of the Ātmā. His every movement, accessory and position is poised to remind us of the Supreme Reality. One needs only to concentrate with awareness on the various aspects of Dakṣiṇāmūrti to gain insight into the authentic nature of Saguṇa Brāhman or the form of the Divine. May Dakṣiṇāmūrti bless us that after having realized his nature with form, we can find rapt audience with Nirguṇa Brāhman, the universal macrocosmic form of God, the infinite and limitless Oneness of all. May Dakṣiṇāmūrti bless us to have the knowledge of that budding cherry blossom of the Self ever at the forefront of our beings.

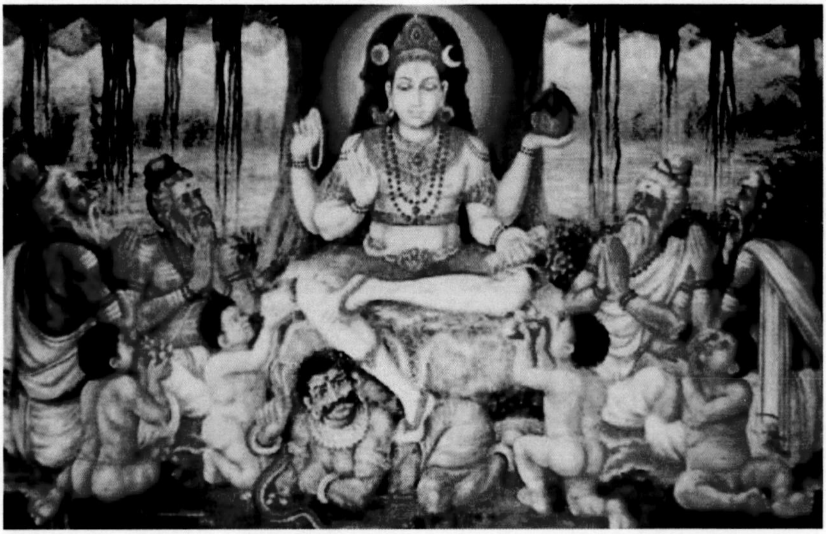

Chapter One

~

THE FOUNDATION

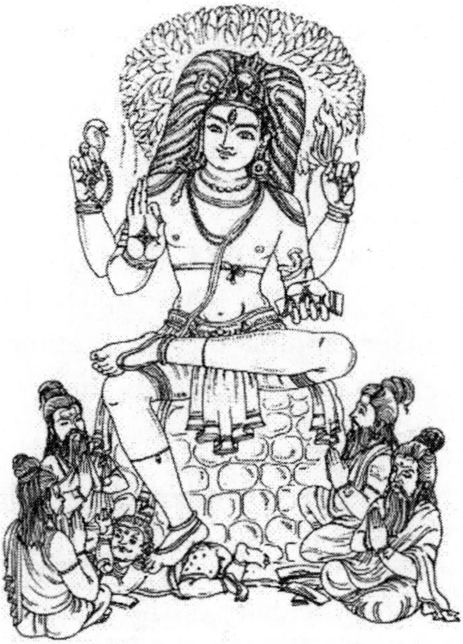

Elements of Kālāmṛta

This updated section explains how to use the information in Kālāmṛta, including the astrological data listed, on a daily basis. General observances for a given day can be made by consulting the tables in the 'Kālāmṛta Toolbox'. Use 'Elements of Kālāmṛta' to familiarize yourself with the astrological elements presented in the almanac and then reference the tables on pages 13 - 19 to understand the basic meanings of astrological phenomena on a given day.

The foundations of most traditional methods of timekeeping are the equinoxes and solstices, as they are heralds of a new season. Notice that Kālāmṛta is still divided into four quarters, in sync with the cornerstones of time however new this year, we make the division as close to the end of the calendar month as possible, still preserving the week in it's entirety. We mark the beginning of each of the four seasons, as defined by the equinoxes and solstices, with a set of the following articles:

1. Dakṣiṇāmūrti: Each year, Kālāmṛta celebrates a deity. This year, we honor the God, Lord Dakṣiṇāmūrti.

2. A two-part series on Palmistry includes both "Understanding the hand types" as well as "Understanding the Lines of the Palm."

Kālāmṛta Toolbox : Beginning on page 36 we offer explanations for the daily astrological data in Kālāmṛta. These updated and expanded tables will assist you in understanding the implications of various Tithis, Nakṣatras, etc., as well as the activities they support.

Pronunciation Guide: On page 241. This guide demonstrates how to properly pronounce the Sanskrit words listed in Kālāmṛta.

The 108 Names of Dakṣiṇāmūrti: On page 228. As always, here are the 108 names in Sanskrit for the deity of the year, complete with proper transliteration and English translation.

Glossary: On page 242. The glossary lists every Sanskrit word, including the holidays, used in Kālāmṛta.

Elements of a Daily Listing

VEDIC MONTHS

Many people who use Kālāmṛta do so for the purpose of knowing when to celebrate holidays, both Vedic as well as Western. Although figuring out precisely when a particular holiday will occur can be quite difficult, some holidays are a bit easier to determine, especially if you know in which month the particular holiday occurs in. For this reason, we include the Indian month on the daily listings. The Indian months are the blending of both the solar and the lunar calendar. Whereas the Gregorian calendar is determined by arithmetical calculations, the Indian soli-lunar calendar is reckoned from astronomical occurrences. So for example, Vaiśākha, the first month of the soli-lunar calendar, begins when the Sun transits into Aries and therefore, the full Moon which will occur in that month will be closest to the Nakṣatra Viśākhā. As you can see, the months are named after the Nakṣatra that the full moon will be nearest to in any given month. Because these months track the Sun's path through each of the twelve Rāśis (signs), there are 12 months. Please see the following table for their names.

Vaiśākha	April/May	Kārtika	October/ November
Jyaiṣṭha	May/June	Agrahāyaṇa	November/ December
Āṣhāḍha	June/July	Pauṣa	December/ January
Śrāvaṇa	July/August	Māgha	January/ February
Bhādra	August/ September	Phalguṇa	February/March
Aśviṇa	September/ October	Caitra	March/April

VĀRA

This element of the calendar is familiar to everyone, as it is used in both Eastern and Western calendric traditions. Vāra is simply the solar day. There are seven solar days of the week, each named after the seven visible planets. The Vāra commences with the Sunrise, not Midnight as we are accustomed to. So a Vāra starts at Sunrise and ends the next Sunrise day. For example, if on the Gregorian calendar it is Wednesday – having changed from being Tuesday at 12:00 midnight – it is not actually Wednesday on the Indian calendar until the Sun rises and makes a new day. The table below lists the corresponding planets general meanings for each day.

Planet	Day	Sanskrit Name
Sun	Sunday	Sūrya Vāra
Monday	Moon	Candra Vāra
Mars	Tuesday	Mangal Vāra
Mercury	Wednesday	Budha Vāra
Jupiter	Thursday	Guru Vāra
Venus	Friday	Śukla Vāra
Saturn	Saturday	Śani Vāra

PAKṢA

Pakṣa refers to a fifteen-day phase of the Moon. There are two Pakṣas within the cycle of thirty lunar days. You may remember that a lunar day is known as a *Tithi.* This is further explained below. There are two Pakṣas — Śukla Pakṣa and Kṛṣṇa Pakṣa. Because Śukla means "bright", Śukla Pakṣa begins with the New Moon and ends with the bright, Full Moon. Śukla Pakṣa is where the Moon is waxing or growing *brighter*. Similarly, as Kṛṣṇa means "dark", Kṛṣṇa Pakṣa begins with the Full Moon and ends with the dark New Moon. Kṛṣṇa Pakṣa the waning phase of the Moon where the Moon is growing more "Kṛṣṇa" or *darker*.

TITHI - LUNAR DAY

A Tithi is simply a lunar day. Essentially, a Tithi measures how far the Moon has moved from the Sun on a daily basis. The lunar months in this calendar start with the New Moon – the first Tithi of Śukla Pakṣa. The waxing Moon cycle – Śukla Pakṣa – is then divided into 15 Tithis, ending on the full Moon. This ending Tithi is known as Pūrṇimā. Then the waning Moon cycle, Kṛṣṇa Pakṣa, beginning with the Full Moon, ends with Amāvāsya, the name of the New Moon Tithi. This completes one lunar month. Tithi names are generally numerical. For example, the Sanskrit name for 'second' is Dvitīyā. The second Tithi would thus be named Śukla Dvitīyā or Kṛṣṇa Dvitīyā. The exceptions to this rule is the last Tithi in each Pakṣa; these have different names. Kṛṣṇa pakṣa, where the Moon grows *darker*, concludes with Amāvāsya. Śukla Pakṣa, where the Moon is growing *brighter*, culminates with Pūrṇīmā, the lunar day on which the Moon approaches the peak of fullness.

Calculating Tithis varies slightly in the different regions of in India. Some assign the Tithi of the day to be the one present at Sunrise. Others consider use the "live" Tithi which can be calculated at any given moment, irrespective of which Tithi prevailed at Sunrise. Kālāmṛta accounts for the Tithis as they occur throughout the day, instead of fixing a Tithi to Sunrise for the entire day. Furthermore, Tithis vary in length from around 20 to 26 hours, depending on the varying speed of the Moon. This calculation is based on the Moon's distance from the Sun at 12-degree increments. Please refer to the next page for a list of the names of the Tithis.

Names of Tithis		
Śukla Pakṣa		Kṛṣṇa Pakṣa
Pratipad	1st	Pratipad
Dvitīyā	2n d	Dvitīyā
Tṛtīya	3rd	Tṛtīya
Caturthī	4th	Caturthī
Pañcamī	5th	Pañcamī
Ṣaṣṭhī	6th	Ṣaṣṭhī
Saptamī	7th	Saptamī
Aṣṭamī	8th	Aṣṭamī
Navamī	9th	Navamī
Daśamī	10th	Daśamī
Ekādaśī	11th	Ekādaśī
Dvadaśī	12th	Dvadaśī
Trayodaśī	13th	Trayodaśī
Caturdaśī	14th	Caturdaśī
Pūrṇīmā (Full Moon)	15th	Āmāvāsya (New Moon)

NAKṢATRA - STAR

LUNAR CONSTELLATION

Nakṣatras (also called stars, asterisms or lunar mansions) historically predate Rāśis (the 12 zodiacal constellations) in Jyotiṣa. Nakṣatras help to demarcate specific portions along the Moon's path through the heavens. A Nakṣatra may be comprised of one star or a tightly clustered group of stars. Using a scheme of 27 Nakṣatras, each one represents approximates the distance covered by one day's passage of the Moon. The Moon takes just over 27 days to complete one circuit of the heavens and return to the same Nakṣatra. Just as opinions vary with regards to determining the Tithi for the day, so too it is for Nakṣatra. Some recognize the Nakṣatra at Sunrise, while others account for the Nakṣatra that the Moon is "in" at an actual time. Nakṣatras almost always change on a daily basis. Kālāmṛta lists these daily changes.

The Twenty-Seven Nakṣatras		
1) Aśvinī	10) Maghā	19) Mūla
2) Bharaṇī	11) Pūrva Phalgunī	20) Pūrvāṣāḍhā
3) Kṛttikā	12) Uttara Phalgunī	21) Uttarāṣāḍhā
4) Rohinī	13) Hasta	22) Śravaṇa
5) Mṛgaśīrṣa	14) Citrā	23) Dhaniṣṭhā
6) Ārdrā	15) Svāti	24) Śatabhiṣā
7) Punarvasu	16) Viśākhā	25) Pūrva Bhādrapadā
8) Puṣyā	17) Anurādhā	26) Uttara Bhādrapadā
9) Āśleṣā	18) Jyeṣṭhā	27) Revatī

YOGA AND KARAṆA

This year we have begun to include the other two members of the Pañcāṅga – Yoga and Karaṇa. While we plan to elaborate on their use in next year's edition, making them more accessible to all, we wanted to include them this year, for those who are proficient with their application. On the two proceeding pages are lists of Karaṇas, Yogas and their corresponding deity. Karaṇas and Yogas always follow the order listed in the tables.

A note on Karaṇa: A Karaṇa is half of a Tithi. While its use in Muhūrta is most important and at times complex, a simple rule for the novice is this: When possible, try to *avoid* inaugurating an important event while Viṣṭi Karaṇa is active. This becomes all the more important if you have a confluence of other negative aspects to the inaugural moment – Say for example, Rāhu Kālam *and* Viṣṭi Karaṇa are active. If possible definitely try to delay or reschedule the start of an important event. Remember, the purpose of Muhūrta and a Pañcāṅga is not to "hide under a rock" during bad times – rather simply inaugurate an event during a time that is as prone to success as posssible. Remember the axiom in the Vedic tradition: A good start gives a good finish.

Karaṇa						
1st Karaṇa	2nd Karaṇa	Kṛṣṇa Pakṣa	#	Śukla Pakṣa	1st Karaṇa	2nd Karaṇa
Bālava	Kaulava	Pratipadā	1	Pratipadā	Kiṃsthughna	Bava
Taitila	Gara	Dvitīyā	2	Dvitīyā	Bālava	Kaulava
Vanija	Viṣṭi	Tritīyā	3	Tritīyā	Taitila	Gara
Bava	Bālava	Catūrthī	4	Catūrthī	Vanija	Viṣṭi
Kaulava	Taitila	Pañcamī	5	Pañcamī	Bava	Bālava
Gara	Vanija	Ṣaṣṭhī	6	Ṣaṣṭhī	Kaulava	Taitila
Viṣṭi	Bava	Saptamī	7	Saptamī	Gara	Vanija
Bālava	Kaulava	Aṣṭamī	8	Aṣṭamī	Viṣṭi	Bava
Taitila	Gara	Navamī	9	Navamī	Bālava	Kaulava
Vanija	Viṣṭi	Daśāmī	10	Daśāmī	Taitila	Gara
Bava	Bālava	Ekādaśī	11	Ekādaśī	Vanija	Viṣṭi
Kaulava	Taitila	Dvādaśī	12	Dvādaśī	Bava	Bālava
Gara	Vanija	Trayodaśī	13	Trayodaśī	Kaulava	Taitila
Viṣṭi	Śakuni	Caturdaśī	14	Caturdaśī	Gara	Vanija
Catuṣpada	Nāga	Āmāvasyā	15	Pūrṇimā	Viṣṭi	Bava
1st K = 6°	2nd K = 6°	1 Tithi = 12°			1st K = 6°	2nd K = 6°

Nitya Yoga	Deity
Viṣkambha	Yama
Prīti	Viṣṇu
Āyuṣman	Candramā
Saubhāgya	Brahmā
Śobhana	Bṛhaspati
Atigaṇḍa	Candramā
Sukarmā	Indra
Dhṛti	Jala
Śūla	Sarpa
Gaṇḍa	Agni
Vṛddhi	Sūrya
Dhruva	Bhūmi
Vyāghāta	Vāyu
Harṣana	Bhaga
Vajra	Karuṇa
Siddhi	Gaṇapati
Vyatīpāta	Rudra
Varīyan	Kubera
Parigha	Viṣvakarma
Śiva	Mitra
Siddha	Kārtikeya
Sādhya	Sāvitrī
Śubha	Lakṣmī
Śukla	Pārvatī
Brahma	Aśvinī Kumāra
Mahendra	Pitṛ
Vaidhṛti	Diti

RĀHU KĀLAM

Rāhu Kālam is a traditional component of some Pañcāṅgams, especially in South India. It is considered an inauspicious time to begin endeavors. In Sanskrit it is said "Upakrāma Upasamharaiyaṃ" that is *what starts well shall end well.* So in practical application, one should not start a long journey during Rāhu Kālam nor should one buy a car during Rāhu Kālam. This is not to say that one should hide under a rock during Rāhu Kālam, rather just avoid beginning a *new* thing during this time like starting a new job for the first day on Rāhu Kālam. It is calculated based on the duration of the day from Sunrise to Sunset, which naturally changes considerably from town to town and season to season. In order to accurately calculate Rāhu Kālaṃ, one must ascertain the time of Sunrise in one's locale. We provide the specific timing of Rāhu Kālaṃ for San Ramon, California. Please refer to www.kalamrita.com to find links your location's specific Rāhu Kālam.

ADJUSTING FOR TIME ZONE AND SUNRISE

An important thing to note is that you cannot use Kālāmṛta without adjusting for the time zone in your locality. Note the time of Sunrise in your locale. Rāhu Kālaṃ is calculated based on Sunrise. Ideally, we would print Kālāmṛta for every place on earth, so each locale would have its own calculations. As this is not practical, users need to account for their time zone and Sunrise time. If you are not in the San Ramon, California area we encourage you to visit www.kalamrita.com for links to region specific Rāhu Kāla timings.

SIDEREAL VS TROPICAL ZODIACS

Kālāmṛta is a mapping of time using the sidereal zodiac - the Nirāyaṇa Cakra. Those familiar with Western astrological calendars will find recognizable elements here, including the phases of the Moon, and many other features of an ephemeris. However, this calendar is based on sidereal placements of the planets, not tropical placements, as Western astrological calendars are.

Although there is only one ecliptic (the path of the Sun), there are two ways to track the movement of an object along it. The first is known as the tropical zodiac. The second is the sidereal zodiac. Note that there really is only one zodiac. The zodiac can be defined as a band, which extends about eight degrees both North and South of the Sun's path on the ecliptic. The 12 portions of both the sidereal and tropical zodiacs have the same names, e.g., Aries, Taurus, etc.

The main difference between the tropical and sidereal zodiacs is in their respective points of origination. The tropical zodiac fixes its starting point on the vernal equinox, while the sidereal zodiac determines its origination point based on the degree of various stars. The difference in the two tracking methods is due to earth's bulge, which causes the globe to wobble on its axis. As a result, it causes the place where the apparent spring equinox occurs to slowly drift backward through the zodiac in relation to the backdrop of the fixed stars.

At one point in time, both zodiacs coincided. However, a phenomenon known as 'the precession of the equinoxes,' causes the two zodiacs to continually move farther apart at the extremely slow rate of about 50 minutes per year.

Currently, the zodiacs are approximately 24 degrees apart from one another. That difference is called the Ayanāṃśa. This means that in one's Western horoscope if the Sun was at 17 degrees Sagittarius, then due to slippage between the two zodiacs, that same Sun appears at 23 degrees Scorpio in the Vedic horoscope.

Using Kālāmṛta

HOW TO USE THE DAILY LISTINGS

This calendar is set for San Ramon, California. All timings are given for the Pacific Time Zone. If your location is not in the Pacific Time Zone, please adjust all times accordingly. Daylight Savings has been calculated into the listings. To use Kālāmṛta outside of the US, please add or subtract the time zone, including Daylight Savings, as appropriate. It is also important to use the time zone you are currently located in when you are consulting Kālāmṛta, not that of your birthplace.

Notice that there are two columns of times listed on a given day. The first column is used only for the beginning times for Rāhu Kālam. The second column lists everything else, including the ending times of the Nakṣatra, Tithi and Rāhu Kālam. The entry times of planets into a new sign are also listed in the second column. For example, on July 4TH this year, the Nakṣatra Kṛttika ENDS at 10:32. The same is true for the Tithi Dvadaśī which ENDS at 16:48. Be sure to note that Tithi and Nakṣatra times are always listed as *ending* times. Also on the 4TH, Mars ENTERS the sign of Gemini at 12:42. All holidays will always be listed on the bottom right hand corner. Note that Kālāmṛta lists the 4th of July - Independence Day - on this day as well.

July			Jyaiṣṭha
Thursday 4			
Kṛttikā		**10:32**	
K 12		16:48	
Śūla		12:41	
Taitila		16:48	
Gara		Full Night	
Rāhu Kālam	15:02	- 16:52	
Mars: Gemini		12:42	Independence Day

Lunar Month: the name of the current lunar month - Jyaiṣṭha

Nakṣatra: the star that the Moon is closest to, here Kṛttikā. The Moon leaves Kṛttikā (and enters Rohinī) at the time indicated: **10:32** (Kṛttikā *ends* at the time indicated)

Tithi: the phase of the Moon: K = Kṛṣṇa or the *darkening, waning* phase of the Moon. Ś = Śukla or the *brightening, waxing* phase. "K 12" is 12 days into the waning Moon cycle. The time indicated is the time that the Moon finishes the listed phase and moves in to the next phase.

Karaṇa: 1/2 of a Tithi; ending time is listed.

Rāhu Kālam: occurs between 15:02 and 16:52

Mars: enters the constellation of Gemini at 12:42

Moon: if listed, would indicate the sign that it enters as well as the time that it enters that sign.

Holidays: are listed in the bottom right of the daily listing.

If you are not in the Pacific Time Zone, then simply add or subtract your time zone from the time of events given on a particular day. For example, if Jupiter changes signs at 8 p.m. Pacific Time and you are in Michigan, simply add three hours to 8 p.m. to arrive at the time Jupiter changes signs in your locale. Again, it is important to use the time zone you are currently located in when you are consulting Kālāmṛta, not that of your birthplace.

All timings are given in military time to ensure accuracy. Thus, 1 p.m. is 13:00, 11 p.m. is indicated as 23:00, and so forth.

Please note that if an event occurs *after* Midnight but *before* Sunrise the following day, we list it as a time over 24:00. For Example:

Wednesday May 1st has the Yoga **Śubha** ending at '28:46'. This means that Śubha Yoga ends after Midnight on the 1st but before Sunrise on the 2nd - 4 hours and 46 minutes after midnight to be precise! You can see the same occurring with the Karaṇa **Bālava** which ends 4 hours and 14 minutes after Midnight.

Wednesday				
1				
Uttarāṣāḍhā			14:12	
K 7			17:08	
Sādhya			7:24	
Śubha			**28:46**	
Bava			17:08	
Bālava			**28:14**	
Rāhu Kālam	13:05	-	14:48	Beltaine

HOW TO USE THE WEEKLY SUNRISE CHARTS

Provided in each week's spread is an astrological chart cast for Sunrise on Sunday of that week. The following tables explain the layout for these charts. The chart style that is used is the version popular in South India. In this style, the Rāśis (signs) are fixed in each box. They do not vary; therefore, the chart below shows the Rāśis as they will always occur in the charts within Kālāmṛta.

Example chart
from July 4th:

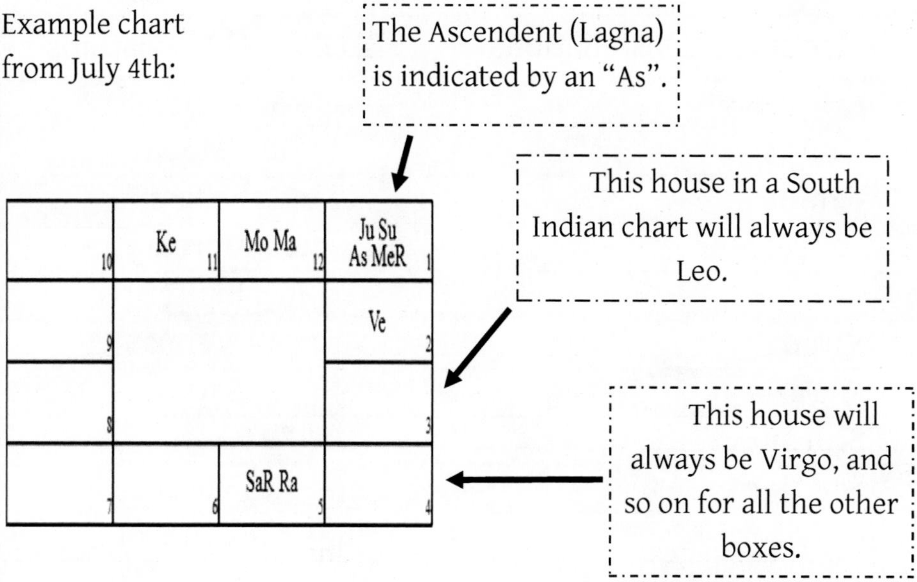

This chart shows how the houses change in relation to the Rāśi (Sign) that becomes the ascendant. The ascendant will always be noted in Kālāmṛta by a '1' and by 'As.' This chart has Aquarius Ascendant:

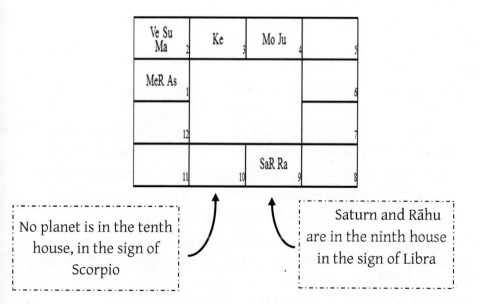

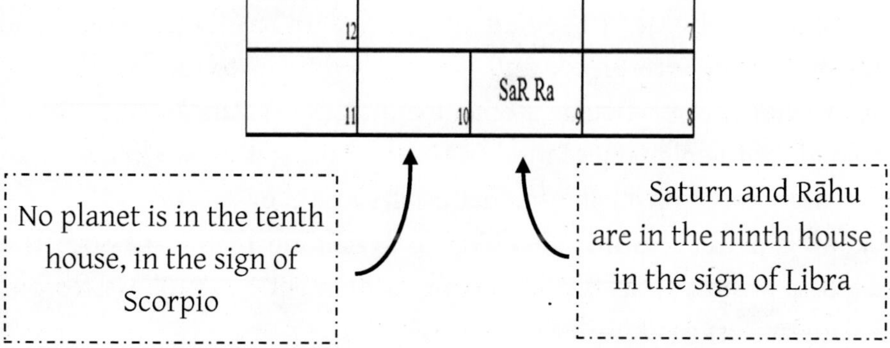

Order of the Constellations	Planetary Abbreviations
Aries	Su = Sun
Taurus	Mo = Moon
Gemini	Ma = Mars
Cancer	Me = Mercury
Leo	Ju = Jupiter
Virgo	Ve = Venus
Libra	Sa = Saturn
Scorpio	Ra = Rāhu
Sagittarius	Ke = Ketu
Capricorn	As = Ascendant
Aquarius	
Pisces	

NEW ADDITION TO KĀLĀMṚTA THIS YEAR:

Puṇya Kālam

Like a lotus, fully bloomed in the high, midday sun, there are many wonderful nuances and beautiful subtleties in a Pañcāṅga. One who is familiar with a Pañcāṅga can tell you that no moment in time goes unnoticed by God. Each and every second has its purpose – and therefore, can be interpreted and effectively utilized to receive the very best of what that particular moment indicates. A Pañcāṅga is able to unfold all of the elements found in time for us, so that we know when the heavens are conspiring for material success or for when they are beckoning us to be still. Listening and yielding to the message the heavens transmit to us on a moment-to-moment basis allows for our ultimate success in life.

How can we tell whether a particular time is auspicious or not? To answer that question, we need to pose another question: Auspicious for what? While the task of trying to find the right time for a particular event can be daunting, embedded within the complexities is a refreshingly simple method to determine if the moment under consideration is auspicious. For at its most basic level, the Pañcāṅga tells us that 'now' is either a good time to pursue materialization or 'now' is a better time to pursue spiritualization.

So there we have it! Every 'now' will either be appropriate for materialization or for spiritualization. So we can categorize our actions by asking – 'Is this activity ultimately about materializing or spiritualizing?' By successfully identifying which of the two basic categories a particular action falls, we can then consult an Pañcāṅga to find which time most supports our intended activity. The "proper time" will then dispense a supercharged energy, whereby the entire creation promotes and supports the best outcome for all of our endeavors – depending of course if they are ultimately 'material' or 'spiritual'.

Sometimes, the heavens are encouraging us to pursue material progress. They whisper - "Now is a good time to marry! Now is a good time to start your business! Now is a good time to go to take that needed loan, meet your boss, write the offer! Now! Now!" Other times, the heavens say "Now is a good time to sit in contemplation! Now is a good time to do japa! [Note that japa is, simply put, the repeated recitation of prayer or mantra] Now is a good time to go on a meditation retreat, to meet your teacher! Now! Now is the time to devote to your spiritual progress!" When we heed these two calls – the material and the spiritual ones – our work and material life will be supercharged with a veritable booster rocket and our spiritual activities will become charged with a divine luminosity. That is why we often hear people say to do spiritual practices during 'Brahma Muhūrta' - the 48 minute period just before sunrise and after sunset. It is well known within the Tradition that certain times of day are supercharged for doing spiritual practice. These times are called 'Puṇya Kāla' which means 'Times of Spiritual Merit' and are the best times for pursuing spiritual practice.

A very powerful Puṇya Kāla happens every month when the Sun changes from one sign to another. A pañcāṅga maker calculates the exact moment that the Sun changes signs and then tells when the period of Puṇya Kāla will fall for that month. This is done using a somewhat complicated formula based on the particular sign the Sun transits into as well as the time of the actual transit. For these reasons, Puṇya Kāla will not fall at the same time each month.

It is interesting to note that while this time is considered auspicious for pursuing spiritual practices, conversely, it is considered inauspicious for pursuing worldly gains. So for example, getting married during Puṇya Kāla – an activity that is essentially about materializing – is not a good idea. The same holds true for meeting a prospective client for the first time during Puṇya Kāla. This year, we are noting the timings of Puṇya Kāla in the calendar section of Kālāmṛta – so that those who are interested can explore deepening their alignment with time. A Sanskrit text, the Rājamartānda, states that "the reward sadhāna done on a Saṅkranti (during Puṇya Kāla) is a thousand times more potent than an ordinary day."

You are cordially invited to explore these potent words on your own. Please note the listings of Puṇya Kāla each month, on its appropriate day and make potent use of them.

WHAT IS A PAÑCĀṄGA?

The word Pañcāṅga literally means 'five limbs'. This refers to five ways that the Sun and Moon can show the progression of time based on their movement through the heavens. In India, these five categories have been defined and observed for thousands of years. Though it is possible to observe the passage of time using any celestial object, the Sun and Moon offer the greatest potential for tracking time on a day-to-day basis since they not only move relatively quickly and consistently but they also are the greatest luminaries in the heavens.

The Sun and Moon are indeed the king and queen of the celestial kingdom and their reign extends down to the earthly realm as well. Every living being is born and thrives by their grace – for their light promotes and regulates our very lives. This relationship between the royal pair of luminaries and earthly life is so deeply intertwined that if either ceased to exist, so would we. Without the Sun we would plunge into a dark, barren world where all life would quickly wither and without the Moon our planet and biology would lose the rhythmic regulation that the Moon provides; tides, pregnancy and the earth's rotation would all be dramatically affected.

The ancient sky watchers knew that the key to tracking relatively short intervals of time was in the orbits of the Moon and Sun. Firstly, they noted a day could be defined by the movement of either the Sun or the Moon. A solar day was defined as the period of time between one sunrise to the next - Easy! A lunar day was tracked by the Moon's longitudinal progression from the Sun in twelve degree increments. On average, this progression takes between 19 – 26 hours. This may sound complex but it really isn't – consider this: The ancients realized that the Moon could elegantly track a month in its cyclical dance from new to full to new again. This was then divided into 30 sections – each of which became a lunar day. 30 days x 12 degree increments = the 360 degrees of the sky! Thus, the solar day was named Vāra and lunar day, or Tithi, became the first two of the five limbs.

The third limb comes from the interplay between the luminaries and is called Nitya Yoga, or often just 'Yoga'. Nitya Yoga describes the angular relationship between the Sun and Moon through a standard formula which results in 27 different Yogas, whose duration lasts about a day each .

Four of the five limbs lay emphasis on the Moon's movement who definitely supersedes her royal counterparts' ability to track time. Half of a lunar day is the fourth limb and is called a Karaṇa.

The ancients also observed the movement of the Moon against the backdrop of the stars. This was (and is) used as a means of observing the passage of time. They divided the zodiac into 27 groups of star patterns, called 'Nakṣatras'. Each solar day, the sky watchers would observe which one of these 27 groups the Moon was in. This is the final and yet very important limb of the Pañcāṅga – Nakṣatra.

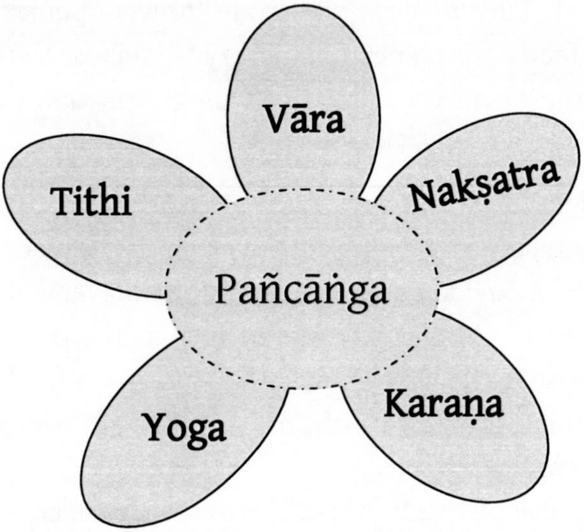

All five limbs were continuously observed on a daily basis and before long, 'Pañcāṅgas' became available to the public for use. These almanacs did not contain only the five limbs but also any celestial occurrence that was deemed relevant for time keeping. Eclipses, the movements of the other planets as well as various other planetary information was also recorded.

Holidays were established when particularly auspicious formations took place as noted through the five limbs. These too were added to the Pañcānga. Over time, a Pañcānga became a household item and today in India, Pañcāṅgas are ubiquitous. The next time you visit India, notice the ornately detailed calendar hanging on the wall of every office and home. Take a closer look and you will see all five limbs listed daily on these modern-day Pañcāṅgas. The tradition of Pañcāṅga use is alive and well in India and now and for the first time, we are introducing it for Westerners in the form of the Kālāmṛta.

Kālāmṛta started several years ago as a hybrid-Pañcāṅga. We included three of the five limbs – Vāra (solar day) Tithi (lunar day) and Nakṣatra. Now, due to popular demand, we are now including all five limbs as well as other aspects of a traditional pañcāṅga, including holidays and astrological articles.

Over the years, the West has integrated some of the very best of what India has to offer: from Yoga to Āyurveda to meditation. Unfortunately, what has yet to be introduced in this transmission is the tradition of time-keeping. Kālāmṛta is dedicated to bridging that gap. The Vedic tradition truly rests on the massive foundation stone of the Pañcāṅga, the steadfast giant who consistently dispenses the wisdom of the proper time for all things, including the daily cycle of the best time to meditate, do Yoga or even administer the treatments and remedies of Āyurveda.

Did you know that Jyotiṣa (Vedic Astrology) is considered to be the 'eye' of the Vedas? The foundation of Jyotiṣa is the Pañcāṅga and without it, the ancients knew we would be lost. All the rituals, so compassionately dispensed in the Vedas to promote peace and prosperity in our lives, would yield tasteless fruit if it wasn't for the spark of ignition that comes with commencing these rituals at the proper time.

Just as we inherently know that eating all of our meals at midnight is not good for us or that planting our garden in the dead of winter won't work, at our core we naturally know how important it is to commence an activity at the right time. However, some of the 'right times' have become unseeable to us, as we have lost touch with our traditions. Working with a Pañcāṅga gives us back that precious sight. By following the daily listings we now can know and even anticipate when it is the right time to do our daily Yoga Āsanas or meditate. We can plan rituals and embark on pilgrimages at the times that are most conducive to do so. We can even use the Pañcāṅga to guide the most mundane aspects of our daily lives elegantly and effortlessly.

There are some things in your life that you can't imagine how you lived without, maybe Yoga, meditation or simply watching the sunrise each morning are a few examples. Trust us, once you begin to use Kālāmṛta, the Pañcāṅga for the West, you won't ever want to go without the incredible sight it brings again!

WHAT IS A MUHŪRTA?

Muhūrta is, very simply put, the formal name given to the process of using astrology to find the most auspicious time to commence an activity. Instead of just choosing a time that is convenient, a well -chosen Muhūrta gives the invaluable opportunity to ensure that one is poised for optimal success. The adage "Good start, good finish" encapsulates the philosophy of Muhūrta.

When we begin an activity at the right moment, it is as if we are dancing in step with the cosmos to the rhythm of celestial music. Have you ever seen someone dance off beat? A bit painful and somewhat amusing, it certainly does not fill the heart with inspiration the way a classically trained dancer can. Watching a professional dancer is mesmerizing. They totally lose themselves to the dance, their body completely surrenders to the music and absorbed in the rhythm, they flow, so graceful, so effortless. We can also dance like this. The celestial music is always playing and just like our dancer, a little training sets us free to lose our selves in the dance.

Setting a Muhūrta can be quite complex and require the assistance of an expert but there are opportunities for even an absolute beginner to select an appropriate time to begin a particular activity. Setting a generalized Muhūrta is easily within your grasp by using Kālāmṛta. A Muhūrta can be as simple as avoiding an inauspicious time.

Say for example you want to apply for a loan and you need to do it on a particular day. Consulting Kālāmṛta and electing not to go for the interview during the inauspicious time period of Rāhu Kālam is a powerful first step into the world of Muhūrta. Like a dancer, begin with just a few basic steps and practice.

In the Vedic tradition, Muhūrtas are set by astrologers for all traditional rites-of-passage, like initiation into learning, marriage or feeding a baby solid food for the first time. Muhūrtas are also set for other major life events, like buying a house or entering it for the first time. Similarly, it is not uncommon to set a Muhūrta for a business venture, pilgrimage or even buying a new car. There are several articles within Kālāmṛta dedicated to showing you how to set your very own Muhūrta, so dive in and enjoy the dance.

Why Should We Use Muhūrta?

The importance that the Vedic tradition places on Muhūrta is immense. For a traditional member of the Vedic society, their entire life would unfold under the rhythmic beat of Muhūrta. Even their conception was chosen according to the merit of the moment. From a baby's first solid food to their first haircut and even initiation into scriptural learning were all done under the auspices of Muhūrta. The society did not live in obeisance to convenience, they lived in harmony with the entire cosmos and that included choosing the proper moment for all important activities. This is half of the reason in which an "arranged marriage" can work exceptionally well, as it has an auspicious time of wedding (along with the husband and wife's birth charts being matched by a competent astrologer, complementing each other in every possible way). This is quite relevant to us today as we are hastened by everything by everything from the constant flow of digital information to the hustle and bustle of daily life. Undoubtedly, as a society, we have lost touch with the natural world around us. Yes, God pervades everything and *is* in the iPod or the Kindle just as much as a blade of grass or a leaf but when we slow down from our fast paced modern lives and act with awareness, the spark of divinity and harmony makes itself known to us a hundredfold more readily. Muhūrta helps us to re-discover our place in that Universal harmony.

One way to understand the importance of Muhūrta is by looking at one of the ancient textbooks of Vedic astrology, *Muhūrta Cintāmaṇī.* Muhūrta Cintāmaṇī begins with a prayer of obeisance to Lord Gaṇeśa. In the author's prayer to Gaṇapati he begs the Elephant-Headed Lord to remove all obstacles that stand in the way of successful completion of his treatise. Consider that setting a Muhūrta as akin to the author worshipping Gaṇapati before commencing his text. Our dear Gaṇapati is the lord of categories and is said that worshipping him before commencing any activity ensures our success. So, the author of Muhūrta Cintāmaṇī begins his text with a prayer to Gaṇapati. "Please bless me in this endeavor. Please let me say what is important and worth mentioning and please bless me to not wander into the unnecessary."

So what does this have to do with describing what Muhūrta is? Think of selecting a proper time to commence an activity, which is what a Muhūrta is, as akin to worshipping Gaṇapati. By choosing the most appropriate moment to commence an activity we are rejecting a multitude of other moments which portend the possibility of obstruction to our intended activity. Choosing to use a Muhūrta is the conscious choice to minimize the obstacles and highlight the benefits of any and every activity.

It should be noted that a properly chosen Muhūrta is not a generalized 'this moment is good' that can be used by one and all. A Muhūrta is a carefully crafted moment that has been chosen by your astrologer for you alone and it is specific for the event you have approached the astrologer about. For example, if you went to your local astrologer and asked them to pick the most auspicious time for starting your new business, they would carefully consider your chart and then after tracking the heavens, would find the best moment for you to formally commence your new business. This does not mean that if you decided that you did not want to start a business after all, that you could now use that moment to buy a new car or get married or that you could sell off the Muhūrta to another entrepreneur to inaugurate their business! Properly categorized, the moment in time was the best for *you* to start your business. Gaṇapati removes obstacles in all of our endeavors and guess what? So does a proper Muhūrta.

Coming back to our example of the astrological text Muhūrta Cintāmaṇī, in the second verse the author tells us that he has composed this book for the success of all rites-of- passage and that success is contingent on knowing when to celebrate these rites. While most of us in the West celebrate relatively few rites-of-passage these days, it is considered vitally important to inaugurate those that we do celebrate at the correct time. That is what a Muhūrta is – commencing important activities at the proper time. A Muhūrta can be used for everything from the first time you approach your beloved all the way to the marriage itself. It can be used to set the time for a big family discussion or giving a family member a loan. Any activity that you deem to be important can be set according to Muhūrta. For big events such as a marriage, starting a business or moving into your new house, it is a good idea to approach a knowledgeable astrologer to help set the date. However, we have created Kālāmṛta to empower you to set your own Muhūrtas for important everyday activities, like meetings or trips. We hope you truly enjoying the dance!

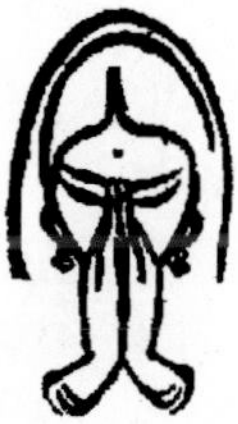

Kālāmṛta Toolbox

TABLES

The expanded and revised table section is one of the most exciting additions to Kālāmṛta this year. We have worked hard to provide you with even more tools and tables to help familiarize you with the attributes of the daily listings in Kālāmṛta. As always, by blending the basic meanings of the day, the Tithi and the Nakṣatra, you can understand the energy of a given day. However, for those of you who want to try to gain even deeper insight into the energy of a given day, we recommend exploring the 'Nitya Yoga' table on page 19, or the newly expanded section 'Nakṣatras and their Qualities' on page 40.

Remember that this almanac should not be used for selecting important Muhūrtas, like a wedding day or when to conceive a child. Kālāmṛta, like Pancāṅga's all over India, provides the data necessary for people to pick the proper moment to initiate daily events in their lives but it does not provide enough information to enable you to successfully set a Muhūrta for big life events. That is because to set a Muhūrta properly it is important to match the elements of a given day to our birth chart. Our birth chart - a crystallization of time - is set from the moment of our birth. All activities we engage in emanate from the potential seen in our chart. Therefore, the moment we choose for commencing an activity should be auspicious both from the vantage point of the chosen time and the birth chart. It is also critically important to choose the correct lagna (rising sign) when considering a Muhūrta for a big event. That does not mean that you can not use Kālāmṛta to set daily activities; we want you to feel confident to use the tools provided to live a more prosperous and successful life, so let us take the following example:

Say that you want to launch a website for your business. You have put a lot of time and effort into building the website and you're banking on the website providing a huge boost to your business. Rather than just launching any old day at any old time, you consult your copy of Kālāṁṛta. Let's say that your webmaster has given you two possible days for the launch. The first step is to look those dates up in the calendar and note all relevant information, just like this:

The first option is Saturday with Ārdrā Nakṣatra and Caturdaśī Tithi in Śukla Pakṣa. The second choice is a Friday with Aśvinī Nakṣatra and Pratipad Tithi in Kṛṣṇa Pakṣa.

The second step is to refer to the tables in this section. Starting with the Saturday option you would note that the Vāra Table on page 38 says that Saturday rules things like labor, work, debt, delay and seclusion. Not really the themes we would want to activate with the start of our website but let's see what Ārdrā Nakṣatra is about. Ārdrā is a Tīkṣna Nakṣatra, and is considered good for all things requiring 'sharpness' in action - hmmm...not exactly the energy needed to launch a website...let's press on and see what the Tithi has in store for us. Caturdaśī in Śukla Pakṣa. According to the 'Tithi Table of Deities and Qualities', Caturdaśī is 'fierce' and the 'Classification of Tithi' Table tells us that Caturdaśī is a 'Rikta' Tithi; empty and hollow. This day is not looking so hot for the prosperity and success that one would hope accompanies the launching of a website. Let's check out the other option, Friday.

The Vāra table on page 14 says Friday is good for wealth and socialization. Well, that sounds promising! What about Aśvinī Nakṣatra? In the 'Nakṣatras and Their Qualities' Table, Aśvinī is listed under the Kṣipra Nakṣatras and it says that on this Nakṣatra it is good to do anything relating to sales! Furthermore, in the newly added 'Sarvārtha Siddhi Yoga Table' we learn that whenever Aśvinī falls on a Friday, this is especially beneficial for the intended activity! Finally, a quick look at Pratipad Tithi, and the choice is clear, for the 'Tithi Table of Deities and Qualities' tells us that Pratipad Tithi has the quality of 'Vṛddhi' (increase) associated with it, and when it occurs during

Kṛṣṇa Pakṣa, it is 'Nandā' which promotes prosperity and happiness, according to the 'Classification of Tithis' Table on page 45.

So the choice is clear, Friday will be the best day to launch the website. A final look back to the date in the calendar tells us that Rāhu Kālam on that day occurs between 10:51 – 12:19. So we tell our webmaster to not launch the site during that time and we are on our way! Easy to do, and well worth the effort! Use this example as your guideline when starting to choose the best day for your intended activity.

Vāra Table	
Vāra	General Meanings
Sunday	King, Government, Temples, Pride, Father, Leadership, Medicine, Victory, Generosity
Monday	Queen, Mental Peace, Agriculture, Mother, Food, Travel, Nurturing, Family
Tuesday	Physical Strength, Battle, Chivalry, Adventure, Passion, Men, Protection
Wednesday	Learning, Intellect, Amusements, Commerce, Communication, Dexterity
Thursday	Advisor, Knowledge, Magnanimity, Reverence, Children Auspicious Acts
Friday	Love, Adornment, Wealth, Arts, Women, Socialization, Advice, Luxury
Saturday	Labor, Work, Debt, Delay, Service, Charity, Old things, Burdens, Decay, Seclusion

DEITY TABLE

As a means of reminding humanity that every aspect of the universe is pervaded with consciousness, the Vedic tradition acknowledges corresponding divine beings for every facet of the cosmos, including the Grahas (planets). The natural outcome of acknowledging the Divine pervading creation—rather than seeing creation as inert - is that one moves through life with respect and humility, constantly acknowledging the crucial role grace plays in bringing the desired fruit to one's actions. The deities listed are numerous, to account for regional differences within India.

Sun	Sūrya	Śivan
Moon	Pārvatī	Śaktī
Mars	Murugan	Hanumān
Mercury	Viṣṇu	Buddha
Jupiter	Bṛhaspati	Guru
Venus	Lakṣmī	Sītā
Saturn	Yama	Kāla
Rāhu	Durgā	
Ketu	Gaṇapati	

LAGNA

The most common way to determine a lagna is by the sign rising on the Eastern horizon for a given time and place. Since the heavens are in motion as perceived from earth, the lagna changes at a set interval based on the degree of latitude of any specific location. Both longitude and latitude are used when fixing a lagna. The lagna is of utmost importance in determining a Muhūrta. Without ascertaining what is the lagna when a Muhūrta is set, as well as the Tithi and Nakṣatra, though the Muhūrta may have thus far been auspicious, it may not be able to yield the promised result. The lagna is commonly called the ascendant or the first house.

SAṄKRĀNTI

When the Sun changes Rāśi (signs) it is referred to as Saṅkrānti. The Sun's Saṅkrānti marks the beginning of a new solar month. This is considered a time to rest, let the new solar energy establish itself, and not undertake any important new projects. Generally, a Muhūrta is not taken twelve hours on either side of the Sun's Saṅkrānti. Refer to the section on Puṇya Kāla on page 26 for more information about the applicable usefulness of a Saṅkrānti. Also, please note that a Saṅkrānti can be applied to the other 8 planets who transit into Nakṣatras as well as into signs.

NAKṢATRAS AND THEIR QUALITIES

This year, we are offering a greatly expanded section of tables on Nakṣatras. This is a very tradition categorization of Nakṣatras which is often used in the setting of Muhūrtas. In this section, Nakṣatras are grouped according to qualities. The quality describes the action that the group of Nakṣatras supports. For example, Sthira Nakṣatras, or 'fixed' Nakṣatras, support actions that one would desire to be of a permanent nature, like planting a garden or laying a foundation. We are also including in the list the Vāra (weekday) which also fits into the appropriate category. Sunday is considered a Sthira Vāra. So if you wanted to plant a garden and you noticed that this weekend a Sthira Nakṣatra fell on a Sunday, then you would want to reserve that day for planting your garden! If you want to get really into it, then consider the inverse – avoid a Sthira Nakṣatra when you are doing an action that you don't want to have a permanent ripple, say, loaning money.

STHIRA NAKṢATRAS (FIXED)

1) Uttara Phalgunī 2) Uttara Āṣāḍhā 3) Uttara Bhādrapadā 4) Rohinī

In these Nakṣatras and on Sunday it is good to do things of a fixed and permanent nature. For example, anything that promotes the longevity of your home, sowing of seeds, planting trees or a garden. Peace or prosperity promoting rituals are also good.

CĀRA NAKṢATRAS (MOVEABLE)

1) Svāti 2) Punarvasu 3) Śravaṇa 4) Dhaniṣṭhā 5) Śatabhiṣā

In these Nakṣatras and on Monday it is good to do anything requiring movement, such as going for a hike, a drive or traveling.

UGRA NAKṢATRAS (FIERCE)

1)Pūrva Phalgunī 2)Pūrva Āṣāḍhā 3)Pūrva Bhādrapadā
4) Bharaṇī 5)Maghā

In these Nakṣatras and on Tuesday it is good to anything requiring ferocity, such as contests, litigations or debating.

MIŚRA NAKṢATRAS (MIXED)

1) Viśākhā 2) Kṛttikā

In these Nakṣatras and on Wednesday it is good to do anything requiring blending or mixing such as the preparation of herbal medicines or tilling your garden. Also, all the things which can be done during an Ugra Nakṣatra can also be done on a Miśra day.

KṢIPRA OR LAGHU NAKṢATRAS (LIGHT)

1) Hasta 2) Aśvinī 3) Puṣya

In these Nakṣatras and on Thursday it is good to do anything relating to sales, romance, learning of sacred knowledge, studying and practicing the arts. Also, all the things which can be done during a Cāra Nakṣatra can also be done on a Kṣipra day.

MṚDU NAKṢATRAS (SOFT)

1) Mṛgaśirṣa 2) Revati 3) Citrā 4) Anurādha

In these Nakṣatras and on Friday it is good to do anything related to learning or music. Buying clothes or wearing them for the first time is also auspicious during Mṛdu Nakṣatras or on Fridays. Playing games, and anything related to friends is also auspicious.

TĪKṢNA NAKṢATRAS (SHARP)

1) Mūla 2) Jyeṣṭhā 3) Ārdrā 4) Āṣleśā

In these Nakṣatras and on the day of Saturday it is considered good for all things requiring 'sharpness' in action.

TITHI TABLE OF DEITIES AND QUALITIES

This table lists the deity that presides over each Tithi, and the general quality of that Tithi. By considering the presiding deity and quality, we can gain insight into the activities that Tithi supports and those it diminishes. The table comes on the page to the right.

Tithi	Deity	Quality
1) Pratipad	Agni	Vṛddhi (increase)
2) Dvitīyā	Brahmā	Maṅgala (auspicious)
3) Tṛtīya	Gaurī	Bala (strength)
4) Caturthī	Gaṇeśa	Khala (contest)
5) Pañcamī	Sarpa	Lakṣmī (prosperity)
6) Ṣaṣṭhī	Ṣanmukha	Yaśas (fame)
7) Saptamī	Sūrya	Mitra (friend)
8) Aṣṭamī	Śivan	Daṇḍa (punishment)
9) Navamī	Durgā	Ugra (fierce)
10) Daśamī	Yama	Saumya (gentle)
11) Ekādaśī	Viśvadeva	Ānanda (pure happiness)
12) Dvadaśī	Viṣṇu	Yaśas (fame)
13) Trayodaśī	Kāmadeva	Jaya (victory)
14) Caturdaśī	Śiva	Ugra (fierce)
15) Pūrṇimā	Full Moon	Saumya (gentle)
30) Amāvāsya	Pitṛ (ancestors)	Pitṛ (ancestors)

SARVĀRTHA SIDDHI YOGA TABLE

This table is a real treat. When looking for a great day to inaugurate or start something, consider trying to find one of the combinations below. Sarvārtha Siddhi suggests that any action done will yield most desirable reward. The combination of a specific Nakṣatra that the Moon is in, falling on a specific day of the week - thus bringing together the perfection of Solar and Lunar energies - was given to humankind out of the infinite compassion of the Ṛṣis. Whether you take this understanding at face value or attempt to dive deeper into the inner significance of the combinations, you surely won't be disappointed! The table comes on the following page.

Sunday	Hasta, Mūla, U. Phalgunī, U. Āṣāḍhā, U. Bhādrapadā, Puṣyā, Aśvinī
Monday	Śravaṇa, Rohinī, Mṛgaśirṣa, Puṣya, Anurādha
Tuesday	Aśvinī, Uttara Bhādrapadā, Kṛttikā, Āśleṣā
Wednesday	Rohinī, Anurādha, Hasta, Kṛttikā, Mṛgiśirṣa
Thursday	Revatī, Anurādha, Aśviṇī, Punarvasu, Puṣya
Friday	Revatī, Anurādha, Aśvinī, Punarvasu, Śravaṇa
Saturday	Śravaṇa, Rohinī, Svāti

CLASSIFICATION OF TITHIS

The following table determines the relative strength of a given Tithi based on the fullness of the Moon. In general, the brighter the Moon, the better it is for initiating a new event, activity or object into use. The following table is an illustration of this simple premise. The Tithis are divided into five categories: Nandā, Bhadrā, Jaya, Riktā and Pūrṇā. Every Tithi falls into one of these five categories. For example, the first Tithi, Prātipad, always falls in the category of Nandā, whether it is Śukla or Kṛṣṇa Pakṣa (waxing or waning Moon cycle). What varies is the auspiciousness of Nandā. This is true for the other four categories based on the phase of the Moon. Furthermore, the five categories are divided into three groups of relative beneficence. When the Moon is brilliant, as would be the case for the eleventh Tithi of Śukla Pakṣa, up until the full Moon, it falls into the camp of 'auspicious.' When the Moon is weak and without light, as would be the case for Śukla Pakṣa Prātipad (the first Tithi of the waxing Moon) up until Pañcamī Tithi in Śukla Pakṣa, then the Moon falls into the 'inauspicious' camp. Use this table to get a sense of the Moon's changing phases and the relative auspiciousness of the Moon on a given day.

Name	**Śukla Pakṣa / Bright Half**			**Kṛṣṇa Pakṣa / Dark Half**		
Nandā	1	6	11	1	6	11
Bhadrā	2	7	12	2	7	12
Jayā	3	8	13	3	8	13
Riktā	4	9	14	4	9	14
Pūrṇā	5	10	15 Pūrṇimā	5	10	15 Āmāvasyā
	Bad	**Neutral**	**Good**	**Good**	**Neutral**	**Bad**

ECLIPSES

"'And on that day,' says the Lord God, 'I will make the Sun go down at noon, and darken the Earth in broad daylight.'" (Amos 8:9)

Astrologers throughout recorded history have recognized the unrivaled power of an eclipse. Indeed, perhaps no event in the heavens has caused as much fear and awe through the ages as a full solar or lunar eclipse. In ancient times, before eclipse cycles were tracked and predictable, the sudden darkening of the sky filled the masses with fear and dread. Even though astrologers have had the ability to predict eclipses for thousands of years, their ability to grip humankind with unmatched fervor has not waned.

Ancient astrological texts offered observers little relief as they unanimously portended great evils for the unlucky land blackened by an eclipse. Whether described as a great dragon eating the Sun and Moon (a view shared by the Chinese and inhabitants of the Indian subcontinent) or as the gods themselves casting darkness over the land (as the Romans believed), most cultures agreed with Ptolemy's great *Tetrabiblos*, which describes eclipses as the "first and most potent" cause of change. To the ancients, an eclipse heralded a sudden and often disastrous event–one to which rulers and their nations were the most vulnerable.

In almost all lands, a ruler kept an astrologer in his court, and one of the star watcher's main duties was to alert the king of impending astronomical omens, like comets and, of course, eclipses. Such an important duty had horrific consequences if neglected. For example, it is said that the infamous Chinese astrologers Hi and Ho were beheaded for failing to alert their Emperor of an impending eclipse.

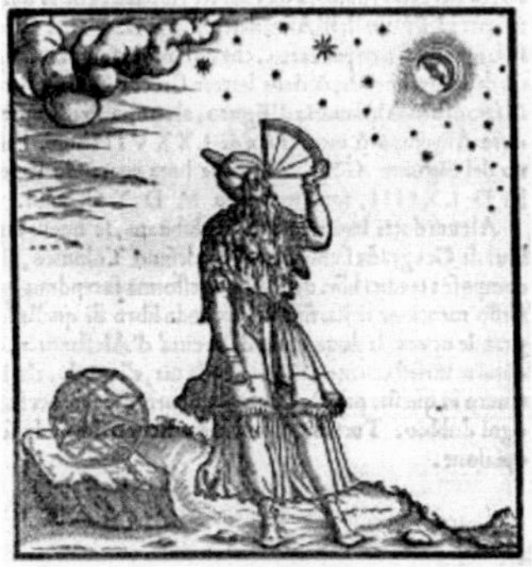

Since the ruler was entrusted with the very safety of his people, his death often meant trial and tribulation for one and all. Thus, every heart filled with dread at the sight of an eclipse, an event that was generally believed to signal a ruler's certain demise. Historically, this was highlighted time and again. In *Paradise Lost*, John Milton wrote:

"In dim eclipse, disastrous twilight sheds; On half the nations and with fear of change and perplexes monarchs"

To protect the nation's ruler, and ultimately ensure the safety of the nation, elaborate rituals were sometimes established. In Babylonia, for example, lunar eclipses were believed to be a particularly evil omen for their kings. So they would appoint a sacrificial king to stand in for the real king during the eclipse. This practice safeguarded the real king while the substitute king was killed, ensuring the accuracy of the omen. Sometimes, kings perished after an eclipse in matters not so orchestrated. In Europe, Charlemagne's son, Emperor Louis, is reported to have died of fright from the five minutes of totality he witnessed during the eclipse of May 5, 840 AD. As if to prove the disastrous effects of an eclipse, his death heralded three years of national struggle as his sons battled for control of the throne. There is also the case of King Herod who died in the year 4 B.C., shortly after a lunar eclipse. And then, in Luke 23:44, we learn that "darkness came over the whole land until three in the afternoon, while the Sun's light failed" in Jerusalem on the very day that Jesus was crucified. (The type of eclipse that actually accompanied the crucifixion is a matter of debate; nevertheless, it is a compelling example.)

The abnormal, dramatic darkening of the Sun or Moon has been used to foretell the death of kings and kingdoms and more. Eclipses have been seen as harbingers of natural disasters, ranging from earthquakes to plagues. For example, the Black Death that swept over Europe was largely ascribed to the lunar eclipse of 1345.

WHAT IS AN ECLIPSE:

How much importance should we moderns attach to the ancient texts and tales?

Let's start with the word itself. *Eclipse* comes from the ancient Greek noun *ekleipsis*, meaning "abandonment;" this, in turn comes from *ekleipein*, "to forsake a usual place, fail to appear, be eclipsed." The noun *ekleipsis* suggests that the Sun or Moon abandon their normal place in the heavens. In the ancient Western world, this idea plagued the people who truly thought that the Sun and Moon had indeed forsaken them, and that soon their rulers would do the same via an untimely demise. This idea is in great contrast to the Vedic tradition, wherein an eclipse is called (in Sanskrit) a *grahaṇa*, meaning to seize or to grasp, which in no way suggests abandonment. The ancient sky watchers of India understood that the phenomena they were witnessing was a powerful seizing of the sky's luminaries by the nodes of the Moon, and that this event had an incredible grasp over the affairs of humankind.

How is an Eclipse Made?

By definition, an eclipse is an event that occurs when an astronomical object is temporarily obscured, either by passing into the shadow of another body or by having another body pass between it and the viewer. Thus, it is not only the Sun and Moon that can be eclipsed; in fact, any planet or satellite like the Moon can be eclipsed.

Still, the term is most often used to describe eclipses of the Sun

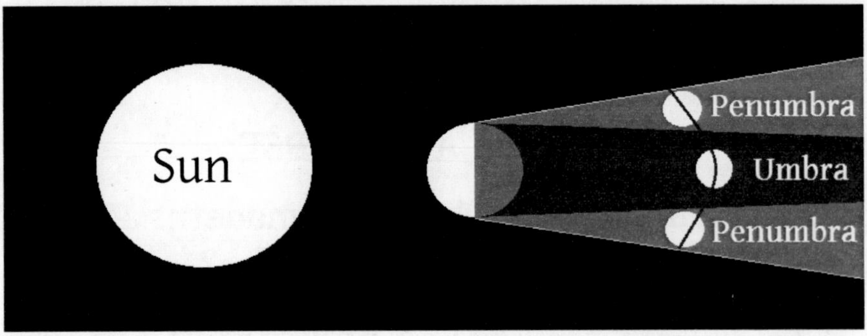

and our Moon. A solar and lunar eclipse both require the Sun, Moon and Earth to be in a straight line so that it appears that one is hidden behind the other as observed from the third.

Lunar Eclipses

A lunar eclipse can only happen during a full moon, when the Earth is between the Sun and Moon and the Earth's shadow thus obscures the light of the Moon. A lunar eclipse is visible from anywhere on the night side of Earth, and while it lasts for several hours, the eclipse's totality (or darkest point) averages between 30 and 60 minutes.

There are three types of lunar eclipses: penumbral, partial and total. A lunar eclipse occurs when the Moon enters the shadow of the Earth, and that shadow can be divided into two distinct cone-shaped parts: the penumbra and umbra. For simplicity's sake, think of the

Earth's umbra as the center of its shadow, blocking all direct sunlight from reaching the Moon; in contrast, the Earth's penumbra is the outer portion of its shadow where the Sun's light is not completely hidden. These two different shadows cause the three different types of lunar eclipses; penumbral, partial and total.

As you might expect, a penumbral eclipse is defined by the Moon passing through the Earth's penumbra (outer portion of its shadow). This type of eclipse is nearly impossible to see because the surface of the Moon is only slightly darkened. A partial lunar eclipse happens when only a portion of the Moon enters the Earth's umbra (center of the Earth's shadow). A total lunar eclipse occurs when the Moon is completely swallowed by the Earth's umbra. During a total lunar eclipse, the Moon passes through all three eclipse types - penumbral, partial and total.

Solar Eclipses

A solar eclipse can only occur during a new Moon. The eclipse is formed when the Sun's light becomes obstructed by the dark Moon passing in front of it, as observed from Earth. As with lunar eclipses, there are three distinct types of solar eclipses; these are: annular, partial and total. An annular solar eclipse happens when a portion of the Sun's surface is visible as a ring surrounding the dark Moon. Partial solar eclipses occur when the Moon's faint outer shadow, its penumbra, blocks a portion of the Sun's light from a specific area on Earth. A total solar eclipse occurs when the Sun's disc is completely obscured by the Moon as a result of the Earth being positioned in the dark center, or umbra, of the Moon's shadow.

Compared to a lunar eclipse, a solar eclipse has an incredibly short duration; even under favorable circumstances, it will not last more than a few minutes. Moreover, a solar eclipse is only visible from a relatively narrow track, called 'the path of totality.' Covering less than 1% of the Earth's entire surface area, this path is typically 10,000 miles long by about 100 miles wide. In order to see the Moon completely eclipse the Sun, you must be somewhere inside this narrow path.

Hybrid Eclipses

Under rare circumstances, a total eclipse can change to an annular eclipse or vice versa along different sections of the eclipse path, due to the curvature of the Earth; this phenomena is known as a hybrid eclipse. There is a hybrid eclipse in 2013.

Eclipse Cycles

Even though we witness both a new and full Moon each month, we don't always see an eclipse. That is because in order for any type of eclipse to occur, several factors must happen simultaneously. Firstly, an eclipse can only occur when the Moon is either full or new, as previously stated. Secondly, the orbiting Moon needs to intersect with the ecliptic — the path of the Sun through the sky, but because of the nature of the Moon's orbit with respect to the ecliptic, this intersection only happens twice a month. Thirdly, an eclipse can only occur if the Moon is either new or full when it intersects with the ecliptic; thus, the Moon will either be with the Sun or directly opposite the Sun on the ecliptic. Finally, even if the Sun and Moon are both at the points of intersection during a full or new Moon, it is not necessarily enough to cause an eclipse. To cause an eclipse of any type, they both need to be within the permissible range of celestial longitude to the intersection points to potentiate an eclipse. If even one of the above conditions is not met, there will not be an eclipse, which explains why it is possible for there to be a full or new Moon near the points of intersection without an eclipse occurring and why we do not have an eclipse every time the Moon is new or full.

Miraculously though, all of these requirements are fulfilled each and every year, resulting in two to three eclipses annually. Moreover, there is actually an 'eclipse season'—a time of the year when eclipses occur. Each eclipse season lasts for approximately 33 days and repeats about every six months, resulting in two full eclipse seasons per year. During the season, the Sun, Moon and Earth align closely enough to potentiate an eclipse; all that is then required is for the Moon to be either new or full. Since the eclipse season is longer than the synodic month (the time it takes the Moon to complete its full cycle of phases, about 29.5 days), the Moon will be new or full at least two and up to three times during each season, causing an eclipse each of those times.

The cyclical nature of eclipses was discovered long ago and the prediction of eclipses became possible through the use of eclipse cycles like the Saros, which was discovered by Chaldeans. If one knows the date and time of an eclipse, it is possible to predict the occurrence of other eclipses using an eclipse cycle. Due to the ability to track eclipses, ancient astronomers have left us with detailed records of eclipses. For example, Chinese historical records of solar eclipses date back over 4,000 years, and have been enormously helpful in measuring changes in the Earth's rate of spin. Thus, the detailed records of eclipses left by ancient astronomers continue to inform modern science.

Sūrya Siddhānta, Bṛhat Saṁhitā & the Vedic Tradition

For those interested in the level of harmony offered by the Vedic tradition, the question naturally arises: What did the ancients of India know about eclipses? Two traditional treatises on astronomy provide the answer. The *Sūrya Siddhānta* is the king of all traditional Indian textbooks on astronomical calculation, supplying astronomical formulas as revealed by the Sun God himself. This treatise is recognized as one of the oldest written records in all of the India canons. Within its pages are three chapters dedicated to eclipse calculation, and so we have evidence that for untold centuries, on a clear Rajasthani night, star-watchers have tracked eclipses. We can also be sure that an eclipse was considered anything but an arbitrary event or even simply an effective means of determining longitude for cities, though they were used for this purpose. The Sanskrit term for eclipse, *grahaṇa*, means 'to seize,' and eclipses were thought to be very powerful omens indeed. The *Bṛhat Saṃhitā*, an ancient, awe-inspiring text by an equally formidable astrologer named Vārāhamihīra, details in verse after verse the potent implications of an eclipse for both individual and nation.

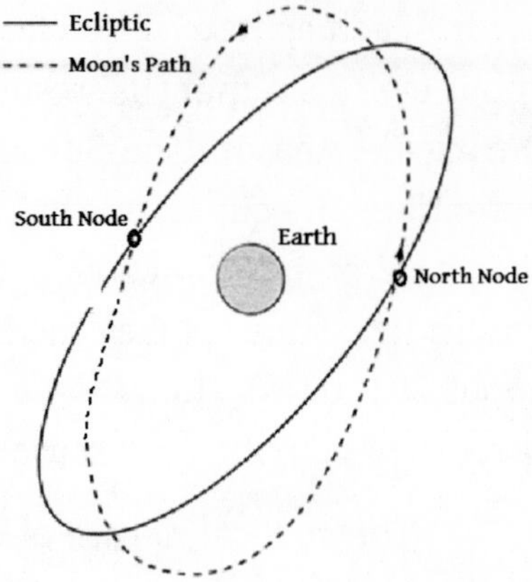

Vārāhamihīra predicts the effects of an eclipse based on numerous factors, including the constellation and astrological house in which an eclipse occurs (there are twelve houses, or divisions of the ecliptic as seen from Earth). It is interesting to note that Vārāhamihīra only mentions the astrological houses above the horizon (houses 1, 12, 11, 10, 9, 8, 7), leaving out any mention of houses below the horizon (houses 2 through 6). This is precisely because an eclipse occurring below the horizon in a given locality is not visible to an observer. This highlights the fact that an astrologer should only be interested in eclipses that are visible in a given locality; we should not attach too much importance to an eclipse that is not visible in our location.

Vārāhamihīra tells us that the house in which an eclipse occurs gives important information about what its effects will be. The constellation, or astrological sign, of the eclipse lends additional meanings. He also informs us that the color of the eclipse and the Sun or Moon's (depending on which is eclipsed) direction when entering and exiting the eclipsed state are determinant. By these means, says Vārāhamihīra, the effects of an eclipse are predictable, but this is no easy task and one best left to the experts (a point he emphasizes). However, he does offer clear and practical advice to the general population by advocating spiritual practices at the time of an eclipse.

These, he writes, will surely ward off any undesirable effects. "It behooves a person to avert the evil effects of an eclipse by japa, gifts, ritual fire ceremonies, and the worship of the Devas and by ceremonial ablutions."

The Vedic tradition is thus aligned with all ancient cultures in correlating eclipses with undesirable consequences. These people of old had an accurate means for predicting eclipses, and a codified way of interpreting them. A vital piece of Vedic culture, in particular, is that it generously and compassionately provides the means for an individual to ward off the adverse effects of an eclipse; specifically, it prescribes performing simple acts of devotion and piety during an eclipse.

The Nodes of the Moon: Rāhu and Ketu

Two important units of astronomical calculation are the two points at which the Moon crosses the ecliptic. These invisible intersections of the Moon's orbit and the ecliptic are called the ascending node or North node and the descending node, or South node. The points are often simply referred to as 'the Moon's nodes.' However, Vedic astrology views these as much more than just mathematical points. Known as 'Rāhu' (North node) and 'Ketu' (South node), these two intersection points are enlivened with a rich mythology.

In brief, Rāhu was a great āsura (non-luminous spiritual entity; a demon) who met his fateful end at a banquet. Rāhu had secretly snuck into this banquet organized by the gods, and had covertly attained the coveted nectar of immortality. The gods' plan was to quaff the nectar in private, at the exclusion of their enemies, the āsuras; however, Rāhu was crafty and powerful; he donned a godly disguise and crashed the party. Just as he tasted the nectar, his true identity was revealed by the Sun and Moon and he was then swiftly beheaded; but it was too late. Some of the eternal, life-giving fluid had already passed into this asura, endowing him with immortality. He now lived on as the head (Rāhu) and tail (Ketu) of a devouring serpent-dragon; opposing ends of the same axis. These immortal troublemakers swore eternal revenge on the Sun and Moon and forever chases them in the heavens; it is said that eclipses occur when Rāhu and Ketu catch the luminaries and steal their light.

Indian astronomers recognized that an eclipse required more than the Sun and Moon meeting at the nodes during a full or new Moon. But the story of Rāhu and Ketu keys a comprehensive understanding of eclipses that incorporates the science of the astronomer with something more. For the Vedic astrologer, the Sun, Moon, Rāhu and Ketu are all *grahas,* or seizers. As opposed to the notion of a planet, or heavenly body, a *graha* grabs on to us, activating our karma (or actions). It is supremely important to note here that a Vedic astrologer does not consider the planets or to use the Sanskrit term, *grahas*, as causal; they do not cause an event to happen. Instead, *grahas* are representative of our past actions, signifying the ripening of our deeds, both good and bad. This also is true for an eclipse. An eclipse does not in itself cause disruption, but is instead viewed as a divinatory symbol; those who know how to read its meaning will gain tremendous insight into events about to unfold.

THE EFFECTS OF ECLIPSES:

What is an Eclipse Good For? Rituals during an Eclipse

It is said that performing any ritual or rite-of-passage during an eclipse should, generally, be strictly avoided. The basic rule of thumb is that pursuing worldly gain at the time of an eclipse is, under most circumstances, contraindicated. 'Worldly gain' here includes anything that promotes one's position or status in the world. This includes activities that would promote your career, health, marriage, etc., and even small daily activities like cooking. Most often, spiritual practices like mantra, japa or meditation are advised at the time of an eclipse.

Vedic astrology is embedded in a deep tradition, one that profoundly contextualizes everything in our experience. Even things that seem inauspicious can become auspicious if we just know how to make use of them. For instance, even though treatise after treatise cautions us not to pursue worldly gain during an eclipse, we are also given stunning examples of supreme auspiciousness signaled by an eclipse. Should this confuse us? Does it mean that the dire warnings should be dismissed?

The tradition is always teaching us, always revealing deep truths, and this instance is no different. Consider this: One of the most powerful instances of an auspicious event unfolding during an eclipse is the birth of Lord Caitanya, which happened during a lunar eclipse. It is said that the local people, upon seeing the eclipse, began chanting, dancing and singing the names of God with such fervent devotion that it deeply touched the Lord's heart and he became manifest on Earth that very night as the incarnation of love and devotion. A jewel embedded within the story of his birth is that in moments of extreme inauspiciousness, (like the eclipse that fell upon the villagers) if we meet the darkening with strength, resolve and commitment to our spiritual growth, (like the villagers devoted singing and chanting) beautiful things will come into existence. Let this example strengthen our faith and resolve.

Periods of 'eclipse' can happen in our own lives, when it seems as though the whole world has gone dark and we are bereft of any light. We may have missed an opportunity or lost something or someone dear to us; but just like the villagers turned to the Lord in their moment of darkness, we should remember the power of taking refuge in God alone—it can surely bring light to even the darkest night.

Through the study of astrology, we gain insight into every moment's purpose under heaven. This is why Jyotiṣa is called the Eye of the Veda. Only by first knowing *what* a particular moment is good for, do we truly have the eyes to see *where* we are going. Without the eyes of Jyotiṣa, life's journey may be more difficult and we will likely run into powerful obstacles along the way; but with the blessing of Jyotiṣical insight, the road is infinitely more navigable.

Eclipses:

Did You Know?

Knowing when an eclipse occurs can be used to your advantage. Consider the case of the one and only Christopher Columbus. On expedition in 1503, he and his men were stranded in Jamaica, where at first, they were treated hospitably. However, after his men cheated the locals, they retaliated by stopping to supply the sailors with food. Ever wily, Columbus consulted his trusted almanac and noted an upcoming lunar eclipse and decided to use that to his advantage. He arranged a meeting with the head chief and told him that his God was angry at the locals for their treatment of Columbus and his men. He told them to observe the rising moon as it would be 'inflamed with wrath', a sure sign of God's displeasure. Moments later, the moon rose, a dark smoky red. The native people were both terrified and amazed, thinking that Columbus must be communing with the Gods to have known such a thing! The son of Columbus, Ferdinand, wrote that the people, " with great howling and lamentation came running from every direction to the ships laden with provisions, praying to the Admiral to intercede with his God on their behalf... " Columbus had one more up his sleeve. Due to his astronomical tables, he also knew when the eclipse would end. He told the leader that God had forgiven them from their misdeeds and his message would be seen in the milky white face of the moon. Soon, the Moon emerged from behind the shadow of the earth and Columbus told the people that they had been forgiven.

Eclipses in 2013

Date	Type	Duration	Area of Visibility
Solar			
May 10 2013	Annular	00:06:03	Australia, NZ, Pacific
November 3 2013	Hybrid	00:01:40	East Americas, South Europe, Africa
Lunar			
April 25 2013	Partial	00:27:15	Europe, Africa, Asia, Australia
May 25 2013	Penumbral		Americas
October 18 2013	Penumbral		Americas, Europe, Africa, Asia

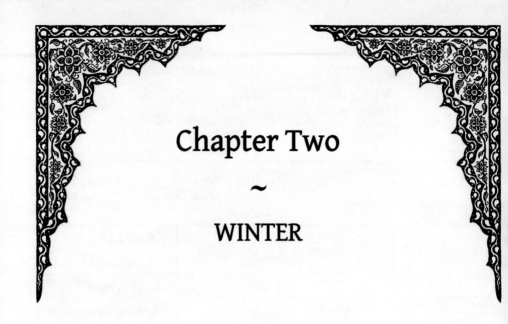

Chapter Two

~

WINTER

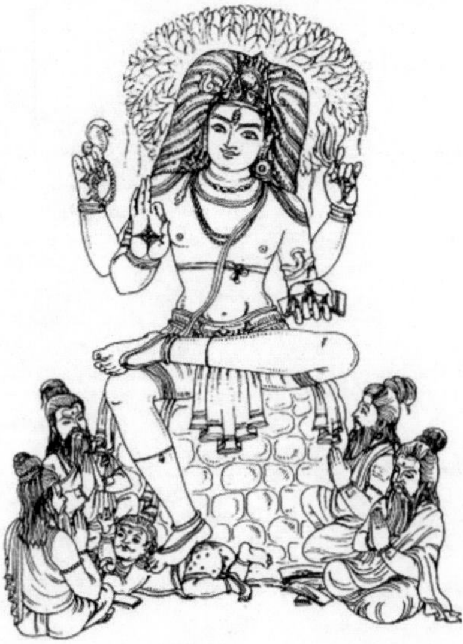

Dakṣiṇāmūrti Stotram: An Introduction

Throughout history, the world has been graced by a few exalted souls that have guided humanity into a deeper understanding with their inherent spiritual nature. These great souls or *mahātmās* have appeared against the backdrop of all religions and belief systems. One of the giants of spirituality that the holy land of India has given birth to is Śrī Śaṅkarācārya. Śrī Śaṅkara was born in the year 788 AD, while India was engulfed in a thick air of religious dogma. Through clean and cutting philosophical debates, Śaṅkarācārya won India back over from the Trojan horse of religious fanaticism.

Along with commentaries on the principle texts of non-dual philosophy, as well as various complementary works on Sanātana Dharma, Śrī Śaṅkara, as he is also known, graced humanity with a text called the Dakṣiṇāmūrti Strotram. A "Stotram" is a spiritual song that is charged with a spiritual luminosity. Stotrams teach the essential message of devotion and non-dual philosophy. Through the spiritual brilliance of a stotram's author, they are often charged with a divine blessing for both their singers and listeners. The Dakṣiṇāmūrti Stotram is one such Stotram, brimming with knowledge and compassion. Please study its meaning and experience singing it daily. The we know that you will not be let down!

Please visit www.kalamrita.com to hear a live rendition of the Dakṣiṇāmūrti Stotram.

Dakṣiṇāmūrti Stotram
Part 1

Mūla Mantra

Oṁ Hrīṁ dakṣiṇāmūrtaye tubhyaṁ vaṭa mūla nivāsine |
Dhyānaika niratāṅgāya namo rudrāya śambhave Hrīṁ Oṁ ||

Oṁ - the sound from which Creation arose; Hrīṁ - the seed syllable that dispels illusion; Dakṣiṇāmūrtaye – He who's form faces the South; Tubhyaṁ - to you; Vaṭa – a banyan tree; Mūla – roots; Nivāsine – residing at; Dhyāna – meditation; Eka – one; Niratāṅgāya – without form; Namo – salutations; Rudrāya – to the fierce One; Śambhave – to the blissful One; Hrīṁ - the seed syllable that dispels illusion; Oṁ

To you Dakṣiṇāmūrti, at the roots of a banyan tree where you reside, meditating deeply on the One Formlessness, you who are both fierce as well as blissful (everything in between is found within you, Dakṣiṇāmūrti).

Dhyānaṁ

Mauna vyākhyā parkaṭita parabrahma tattvaṁ yuvānaṁ
Varṣiṣtha antevasa dṛṣigaṇair āvṛtaṁ brahma niṣṭhaiḥ |
Ācāryendraṁ karakalita cinmudram ānanda rūpaṁ
Svātmārāmaṁ mudita vadanaṁ dakṣiṇāmūrtimīḍe || 1 ||

Mauna – silence; Vyākyā – teaching; Prakaṭita – is revealed; Parabrahma – the Supreme Reality; Tattvaṁ - Truth; Yuvānaṁ - ever youthful; Varṣiṣṭha – old in age; Antevasad –who dwell near the teacher; Ṛṣi – sages; Gaṇaiḥ - a group of; Āvṛtaṁ - surrounded by; Brahmaniṣṭhaiḥ - those committed to Knowledge of the Self

Ācāryendraṁ - the first and foremost teacher; Kara – hand; Kalita – made or done with; Cinmudram – gesture of "Reality"; Ānanda – pure bliss; Rūpaṁ - form of; Svātmā – his very Self; Rāmaṁ - reveling; Mudita – joy; Vadanaṁ - face; Dakṣiṇāmūrti – Him facing South; .Īḍe - I offer respect to

He who is ever youthful is surrounded by a gaggle of aged sages. These sages are committed to the Knowledge of the Self. Dakṣiṇāmūrti is teaching the Supreme Reality to them through the medium of pure silence. This foremost amongst teachers holds his hand in the gesture of divinity and reveling in his essential nature which is the very Self of all, has a deep look of serenity on his face. To Him, I offer my deepest respect.

Intro: Verse 2

Vaṭa viṭapi samīpe bhūmibhāge niṣaṇṇaṁ |
Sakala muni janānāṁ jñāna dātā ramārāt ||

Vaṭa – a banyan tree; Viṭapi – a thicket; Samīpe – proximal to; Bhūmi – earth; Bhāge – a place on; Niṣaṇṇaṁ - sitting; Sakala – all; Muni-janānāṁ – holy people; Jñānadāta – knowledge is given; Aramārāt – openly

Seated under a banyan grove, Dakṣiṇāmūrti gives the Knowledge of the Self to all spiritual seekers and wise-people.

Intro: Verse 3

Tribhuvana gurumīśaṁ dakṣiṇāmūrti devaṁ |
Janana maraṇa duḥkha ccheda dakṣaṁ namāmi ||

Tribhuvana – three worlds; Gurumīśaṁ - teacher of teachers; Dakṣiṇāmūrtidevaṁ - worshipful Dakṣiṇāmūrti; Janana – birth; Maraṇa – death; Duḥkha – suffering; Cheda – fissure; Dakṣaṁ - prompt, alert; Namāmi – I bow to you

Reverent salutation to the worshipful One Facing South who is at the foot of a wide stretching banyan tree. He dispenses Supreme Knowledge by teaching the essence of birth, death and suffering and the inherent distress therein to those fit sages who accompany him.

Intro: Verse 4

Citraṁ vaṭataror mūle vṛddhāḥ śiṣyā guruRyuvā |
Gurostu maunaṁ vyākhyānaṁ śiṣyāstu chinnasaṁśayāḥ ||

Citraṁ - shinning; Vaṭa – banyan tree; Tara – clean; Mule – at the foot of; Vṛddhāḥ - advanced in years; Śiṣyā – students; Guru – teacher; Yuvā – youthful; Gurostu – the teacher is; Maunaṁ - silence; Vyākhyānaṁ - in words of; Śiṣyāstu – student's that are; Chinnasaṁśayāḥ - those who's doubts are dispelled

At the base of a holy banyan tree, a group of aged sages are gathered around an ever youthful teacher who is imparting knowledge to them through the medium of silence. Through this teaching, all doubts are completely dispelled.

Intro: Verse 5

Nidhaye sarva vidyānāṁ bhiṣaje bhāva rogiṇām |
Gurave sarva lokānāṁ dakṣiṇāmūrtaye namaḥ ||

Nidhaye – in the repository; Sarva – all; Vidyānāṁ - knowledge; Bhiṣaje – healer of; Bhavarogiṇām – stigmatism of improper view; Gurave – to the teacher; Sarvalokānāṁ - all of the realms of existence; Dakṣiṇāmūrtaye – who is in that Form; Namaḥ - I salute

Obeisance to Dakṣiṇāmūrti, the holder of all sacred knowledge, who heals those afflicted from the stigmatism of improperly viewing life and is the teacher of all realms of existence.

Intro: Verse 6

Oṁ namaḥ praṇavārthāya śuddha jñānaika mūrtaye |
Nirmalāya praśāntāya dakṣiṇāmūrtaye namaḥ ||

Namaḥ - salutations; Praṇava – the sound *Oṁ*; Arthāya – the source of; Śuddha – pure; Jñānaika – knowledge of the Indivisible; Mūrtaye – in the form of; Nirmalāya – to the blemishes one; Praśāntāya – to the serene one; Dakṣiṇāmūrtaye – in the form of the one facing South; Namaḥ - salutions

Salutations to the pure and serene teacher that is facing South. He holds the knowledge of the One indivisible existence of All and is the essence of the Oṁ mantra.

To be continued...

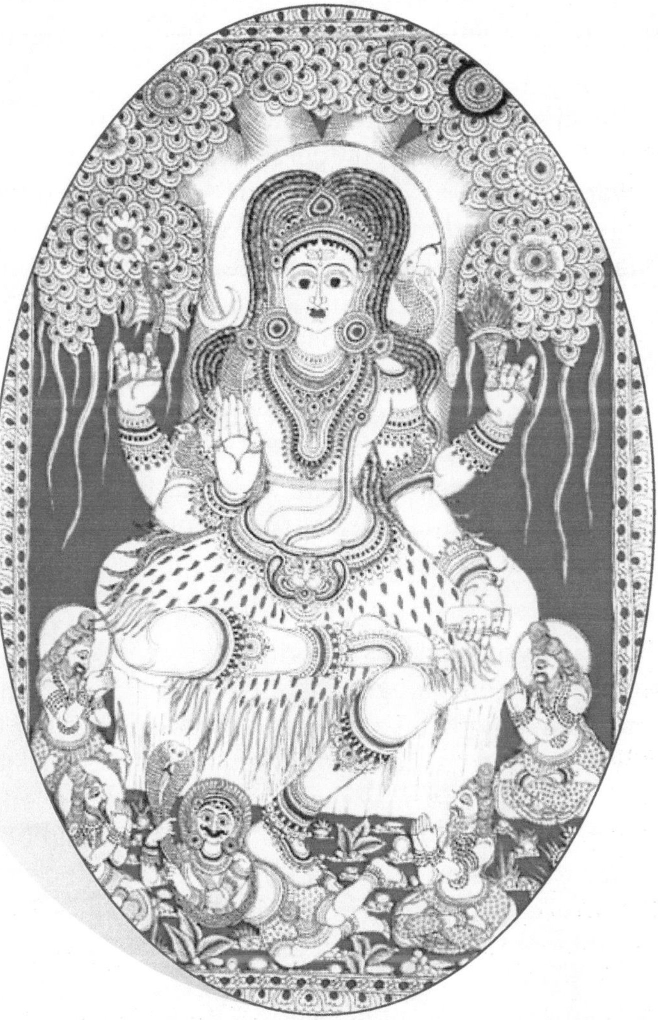

Hasta Sāmudrika Śāstra
~
An Introduction to Vedic Palmistry

Hasta Sāmudrika Śāstra, also known as 'Hasta,' is the ancient Vedic science of hand analysis, or palmistry. In Hasta, the structure of the hand along with its lines and markings are interpreted as symbols that indicate the likely trajectory of one's path in this lifetime. The hand becomes a portent, an omen, of our tendencies, talents, psychology, and all manner of underlying potential.

Hasta gives us a means to access the karmic blueprint that pervades and subtly colors our perceptions and actions. It helps us become aware of how our tendencies and individual filters influence our actions and hence the world around us. This awareness empowers us to influence the interplay between fate and freewill in our lives—the more we are aware of our propensities and strategies, the more we can exercise flexibility in our choices when we interact with our environment. For instance, if I know I have a tendency towards using speech that others often experience as being too harsh, I can use my attention and awareness to make my speech more gentle and kind. Understanding our karmic blueprint allows us to be less reactive, more in tune with our needs and those of the people around us, and gives us greater flexibility of expression in our interactions.

Hand analysis offers us the gift of becoming aware of our own patterns. But it also encourages compassion of others by helping us to understand their unique character as expressed through their hands. Someone with a hand that displays characteristics associated with the fire element, for example, may feel compelled to move on from a task before it is completed. When a person with a fire hand (in contrast to one with an earth, water, or air hand) encounters an obstacle at work or in relationship, impatience may drive them to give everything up. Empowered by the insight of hand analysis, such a person can learn to relax, invoke patience, and remember that there are more productive strategies available than walking away from it all. Likewise, it can give us compassion for what might otherwise be inexplicable actions.

First and foremost, practicing Hasta properly involves the correct understanding and application of a series of principles. Knowing how these principles are categorized is part of the oral tradition of Hasta Sāmudrika Śāstra, and is necessary to the mastery of the subject. Yet you'll be hard-pressed to find discussion of this in print. Have you leafed through a

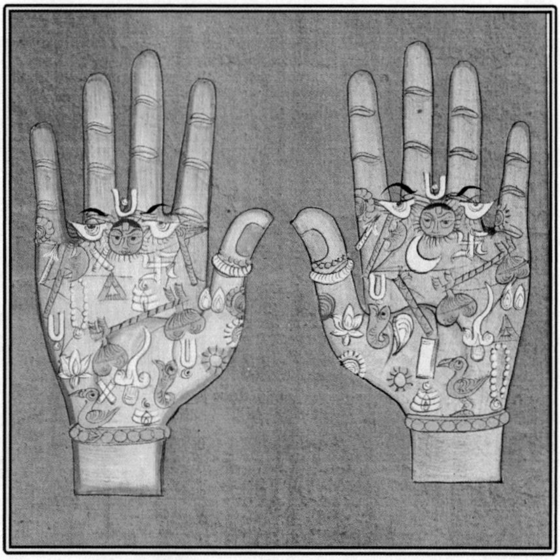

book on palmistry only to be left feeling confused? How are all those individual categories combined into something meaningful? Understanding what features are the strongest indicators of character tendencies is the most potent tool in the Hasta toolbox, and something that we attempt to illustrate in this book.

When examining a person's hands, the tradition instructs us to first assess the overall structure of the hand. Is it a rough, firm, short-fingered, solid earthy hand or an elongated, soft, flexible, long-fingered water hand? Is it the hand of the impetuous fire type or the thoughtful intellectual air type? The overall structure of the hand gives us a solid foundation from which to interpret all of the other details that the hand reveals. Contrary to popular belief, to delve immediately into the lines and markings of a hand glosses over the overall landscape that ultimately contextualizes these details. It is akin to purchasing a house solely because you are enamored with its light fixtures, without taking into consideration the neighborhood the house is in, let alone the solidity of the foundation or the condition of the roof.

Someone with a hand that displays characteristics associated with the fire element, for example, may feel compelled to move on from a task before it is completed. When a person with a fire hand (in contrast to one with an earth, water, or air hand) encounters an obstacle at work or in relationship, impatience may drive them to give everything up. Empowered by the insight of hand analysis, such a person can learn to relax, invoke patience, and remember that there are more productive which we consciously express who we are. At any given point in time, we are infinitely more aware of what our fingers are doing in space than of what our palms are doing.

Though palms vary in dimension, they can be classified as being wide (mostly shaped like a square) or narrow (shaped like a rectangle). Fingers, as measured in relation to the palm, vary from short to long. The wider a palm—the more it gives the impression of a square—the more stable, resistant, pragmatic, and objective the person will be. Those with square palms tend to value common sense and be guided by a strong need for security in their environment. They have strong survival instincts and respond better under pressure than do those with narrower palms. The narrower a palm, the more its shape resembles a rectangle instead of a square. Those with narrow palms are sensitive, idealistic, uncertain, intuitive, and emotional. These meanings come from the natural world, in which a square is a more stable form than a rectangle, the more so when the rectangle becomes overly narrow. A one-story structure, for example, will withstand an earthquake better than a skyscraper, all other things being equal.

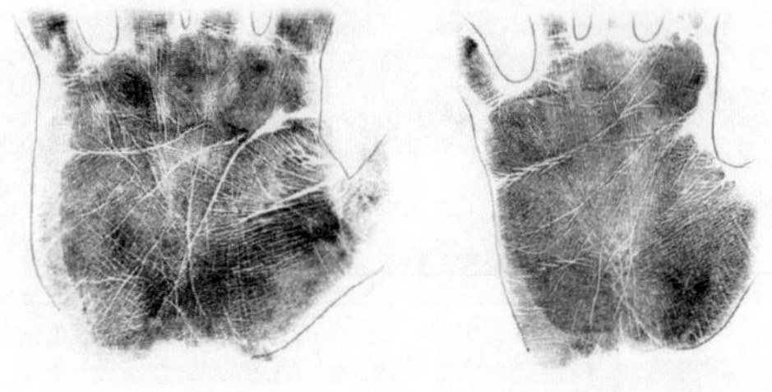

Wide Palm Narrow Palm

Measuring finger length can be a tricky task. A technique used by savvy palmists is to simply 'eyeball' finger length; short fingers just look short! However, they also know that the average length of fingers is about 3/4 of the length of the palm, as measured from the base of the middle finger to the center of the wrist. Please note that the middle finger is the representative for the entire hand's finger length. So, when in doubt, simply measure the middle finger and compare that measurement to the palm's length: is the middle finger less than 3/4 of the length of the palm (denoting short fingers) or greater than 3/4 of the length of the palm (showing long fingers)? Again, if the middle finger is longer than the 3/4 mark, the fingers are long. And vica-versa for short. Please refer to the diagram above for an example of finger lengths. After measuring several hands, you will get the feel for it and will eventually be able to eyeball it like the experts.

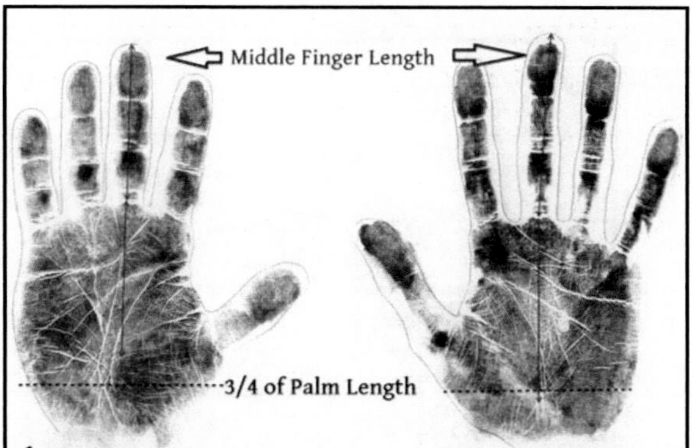

Short Fingers Long Fingers

Now that we know the palm width and finger length, we can determine the basic elemental structure of a person's hands. Does the person have an earth, fire, water or air hand? Diagrams of each elemental type can be found in each Hasta Sāmudrika articles within Kālāmṛta. The combination of rectangular palms with short fingers provides the foundation for the fire hand, for example. What does this mean? It means that the qualities of that particular element are predominant for the person and will often characterize their behaviors. You will be surprised at how much you can learn about an individual simply by being able to recognize which type of hand they have. In the case of the fire hand, the qualities of warmth, sharpness, and mobility are found both in the structure and details of the hand and in the very nature of the person. A person with a fire hand will be 'fiery' in character. They will be friendly, have a quick temper, and will love physical movement.

Once we have determined a person's elemental hand type, we can add the color of detail. We may consider the texture of the skin, the quality of the lines, and the type of fingerprints. But remember that these fascinating details are subordinate to and only properly understood in the context of the overall shape of the hand. Let's say that we find a passionate heart line in a palm; that heart line will express itself in dramatically different ways depending on the type of hand: earth, fire, water or air. More will be revealed in the seasonal articles.

May you enjoy this deep exploration of yourself through the ever changing and evolving mirror of your hands!

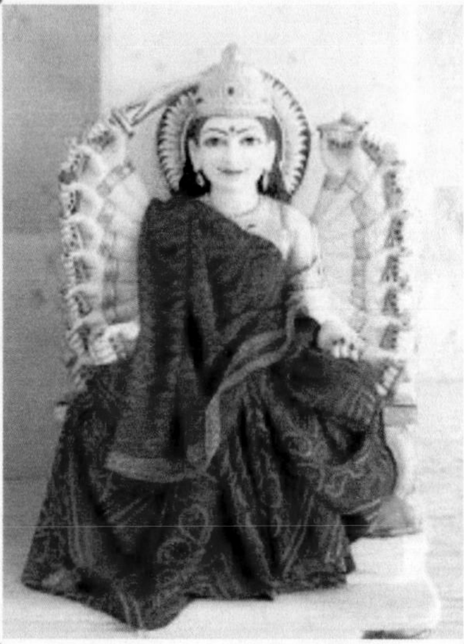

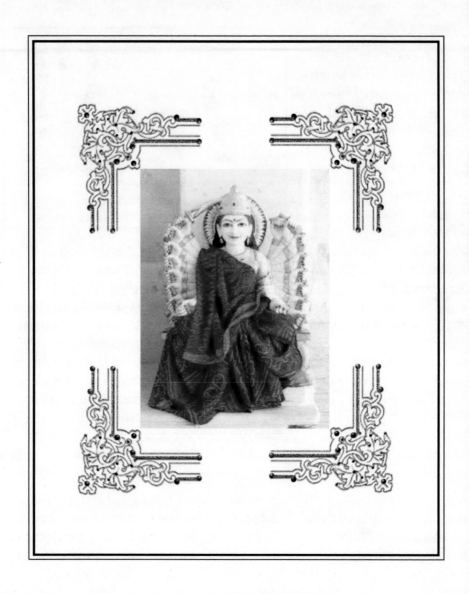

ॐ पञ्चाङ्गुल्यै नमः

Oṃ Pañcāṅgulyai Namaḥ

Salutations to Pañcāṅgulī Devī,
bestower of the knowledge of Hasta Sāmudrika

Hasta Sāmudrika Śāstra

~

The Earth Hand

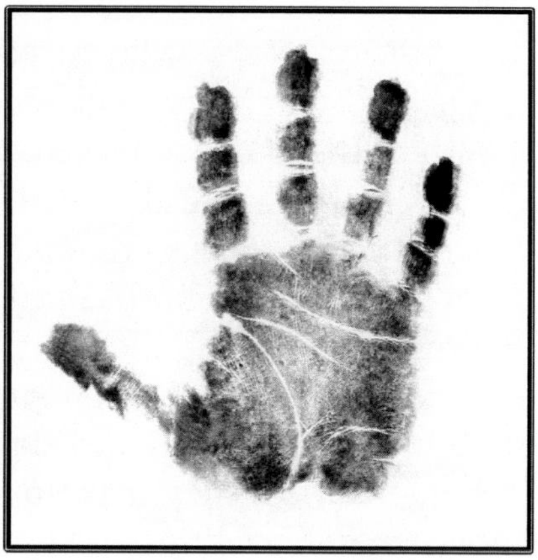

We begin our exploration of hand types with the hands that build our world and till our fields, the hands that are not afraid of hard work and that love the outdoors: the strong hands dominated by the earth element. Earth is cold, solid, heavy, hard, and rigid. These qualities are seen both in the structural characteristics of the hand and in the way an earth handed person relates to his or her environment.

Palm

Earth hands have palms that are mostly square in shape. While a perfect square shape doesn't exist in nature, the palm of an earth hand has a distinctly squarish look as opposed to a long or narrow appearance.

The square palms of an earth hand indicate stability and solidity. These qualities are usually reflected in the person's whole body—earth-handed people are often, compact and resilient, and of all the hand types they are the healthiest and most endowed with natural endurance. They can work hard because their bodies support hard work. Their movements are slow but functional, and they tend to focus on one thing at a time. On an emotional level, the square-palmed stability of the earth hand tends to make these type of people practical and extremely reliable.

In addition to their squarish shape, the palms of an earth hand are often thick and inflexible. This can manifest as a resistance to change. The Earth Hand is the one who shows up at the town meeting to block the new building proposal because they are suspicious of things new and different. Typical earth-handed people favor the tried and true in life.

Fingers

The fingers of an earth hand are relatively short compared to the palm. To determine if fingers are long or short, first measure the length of the palm from the center of the wrist to the base of the middle finger; then measure the length of the middle finger and compare this to the palm measurement. Fingers measuring less than 3/4 of the palm's length are short! Short fingers indicate someone who is more interested in the big picture than in the details. They understand the natural world and its cycles simply and spontaneously, and this understanding makes them appreciate how things fundamentally function as opposed to how they may appear. They are practical-minded, salt-of-the-earth personalities.

Like the palm of an earth hand, the fingers of such a hand tend to be on the inflexible side. To test how flexible the fingers of a hand are, place the hand - palm down - on a flat surface and pick up the fingers. Fingers that barely come off the surface are inflexible and indicate somebody who likes routines and habits and can be quite resistant around change and variety. They don't just accept a new thing for the sake of novelty, but when shown the utility of a new object or idea, they warm up to it.

It can be all too easy to think of earth-handed people as resistant to new opportunities but what if we reframe this notion? What if, instead of viewing the earth-handed person as a veritable "stick-in-the-mud", we understand the value the person places on the reliability, usefulness and dependability of people and things? If we recognize the inherent value standing steadily in the heart of our dear earth-handed friend, we may benefit from their solid, stable point-of-view.

Skin Texture

Earth hands tend to have skin that is rough to the touch. Most people think that skin texture is a result of how we use our hands. For example, a gardener has rougher hands than a computer programmer because gardening is harder on skin than typing. While that is partly true, the inverse might be true as well: those with rougher skin have a more sensory-based nature and are therefore attracted to more practical, hands-on activities. So perhaps it's having the rough skin to begin with that attracts the person to go work in a garden instead of sitting at a desk.

Thick, rough skin goes along with a certain resolute quality that earth-handed people possess. Earth-handed types can be reserved and very matter-of-fact. It's not always easy to make new friends with an earth-handed person mostly because they take comfort in a tight social circle of family, relatives, and people they have known for quite some time. We should all be so lucky as to have an earth-handed person among our family and friends. They are practical, level headed, and supportive.

Lines

Earth hands usually have few lines. In fact, they have fewer lines than any other hand type. Frequently an earth hand displays only the three major lines which are wide and tend not to cross. These clear, simple lines reflect the sensorial and uncomplicated nature of those with these hands. Earth-handed folks relate to their surroundings through their senses. They not only love to be outdoors but also usually prefer living away from the hustle and bustle of city centers. Visit your local farmers' market and you are bound to find some earth-handed people handing you the fruits of the earth that they themselves have harvested.

Fingerprints

Earth hands often have one or more fingers with arch fingerprints. Arch fingerprints look just like an arch or a low wave in the lines that make up the fingerprints. Arch fingerprints, although the simplest pattern amongst fingerprints are also the rarest. In fact, it is highly unusual to see a set of hands

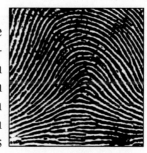

With more than three or four arch fingerprints. Because of their rarity, not all earth hands are going to have arch fingerprints. When they are present, they add to the resourceful, efficient nature of the typical earth-handed person. Arches can also indicate specific manual skills.

Earth and fire hands comprise the majority of hand types on the planet. When we live in a city, we may not fully appreciate that our sustenance largely relies on the honest, hard work of hearty earth hands. We rely on the earth for support, for food and for our very existence. The earth is, above all, productive and beneath its surface there is always a quick ferment of life. Break through the reserve of the earth-handed person - but be careful to not disturb them by probing too deeply! - and you will be pleasantly surprised by their reliability and sense of justice. They are strong providers and well-balanced, nonintellectual, self-possessed, realistic and literally down-to-earth!

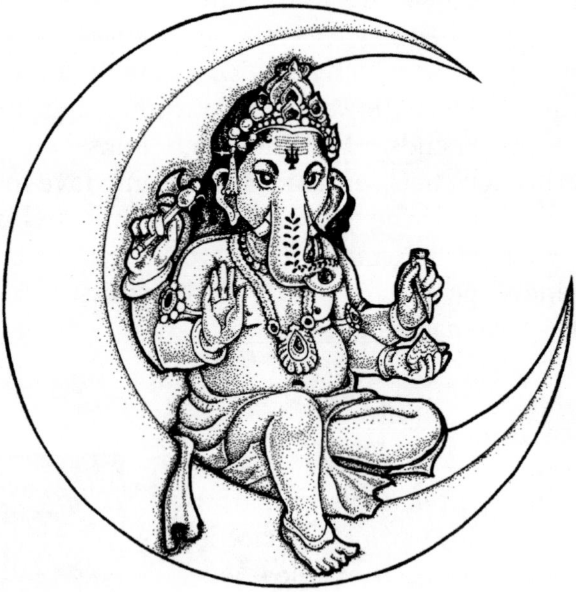

Hasta Sāmudrika Śāstra

~

The Life Line

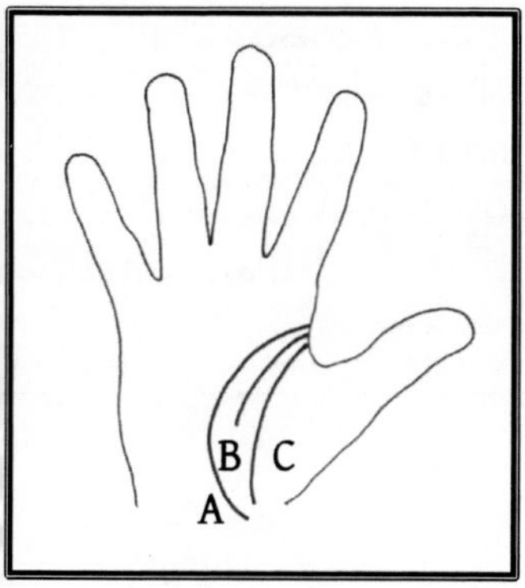

The Life Line is the principle line on the hand. It is found on all hands without exceptions, although variations do occur and occasionally this line can be tricky to identify. Its origin is at the edge of the palm in the area between the thumb and the base of the index finger, and it curves down and around towards the wrist forming an arc around the base of the thumb.

The life line provides information about the amount of life force available to us and how our life force expresses as physical strength, energy level, vitality, and recuperative ability. They do this in a variety of ways. Above, letter *A* represents a long and curved life line; letter *B* shows a straight line and letter *C* shows a narrow and straight line. Let's take a moment now to delve deeper into the meanings of these lines.

This line is also a visible gauge of major happenings in our life, and is heavily used by hand analysts for timing events and obstacles. The part of the line under the index finger represents our early years, and the farther down towards the wrist the later portion of our lives. That is why, for example, in Vedic rituals to honor the ancestors, offerings are made by pouring libations from the palm towards the area between the thumb and the index finger, towards the origin of our life that our ancestors represent.

Length

Life lines can be short or long. Since this line starts between the thumb and index finger and travels towards the wrist, a long life line is going to be one that goes all the way down to the wrist. A short life line, is going to be one that ends somewhere before getting to the wrist. A long life line, provided the line is unblemished, indicates

Life Line Length

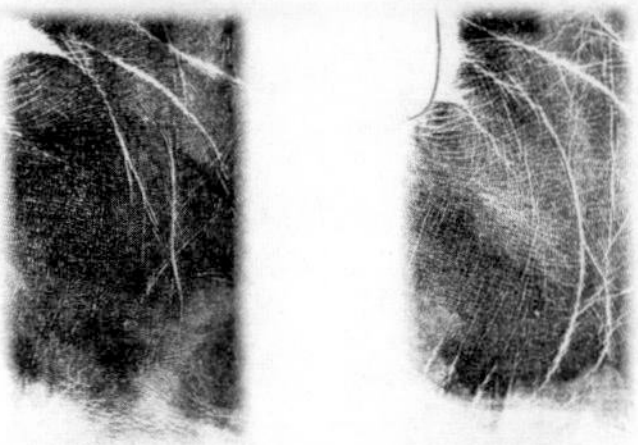

Short Long

someone who has great physical resources available. They possess more stamina and resilience than a short life line. The shorter the line, the less of these qualities, although truly short life lines are rare.

Contrary to popular misconceptions, the length of the life line is not an indicator of longevity. For example, a short life line does not mean that one is destined to live a short life. A short lifeline, though, can be an indicator of the necessity to make health and vitality cultivation a priority.

Curvature

Life Line Curvature

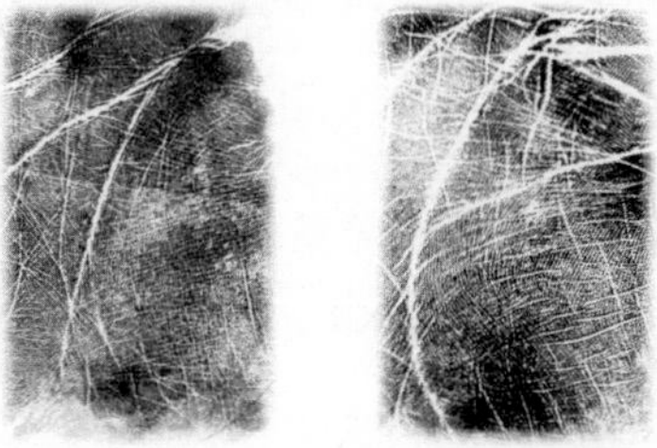

Straight Curved

Life lines have different curvatures, and the arc they form is a visual guide to how much energy is available. The wide-sweeping and curved life line flows out towards the center of the palm, creating a large area at the base of the thumb. This adds health and vitality to the lifeline. These life lines indicate a great enthusiasm for life, a willingness to undertake challenges, and the health and vitality necessary to support much activity. The straighter life line, instead, tightly hugs the ball of the thumb. This can be a sign of reduced endurance and a delicate constitution.

Quality

In general, the stronger a line, the more the characteristics associated with that line express in the life of the person. If you have a well-marked, clear, strong life line you can expect to have reasonably good physical health, vitality, and resilience.

Lines are conduits of energy and as such we like them to be strong, clear, unobstructed, deep and thick so that the energy that they represent flows powerfully and without obstacles. The stronger the lifeline, the greater the life force. This energy is going to seek expression through physical activity and endurance. For example, athletes have more prominent and powerful life lines than intellectual thinking types.

Life Line Quality

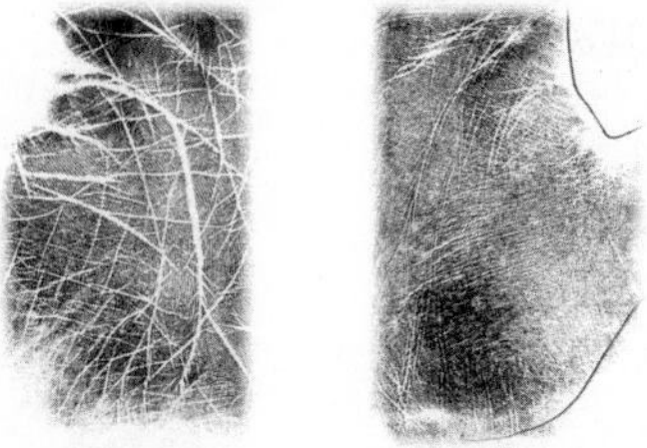

Strong **Weak**

The stronger the line, the stronger and healthier the person is in general. Having a strong life line does not mean that one is not subject to occasional ill health, but it does indicate a stronger constitution and a greater capacity to recover from illness and injury.

A weaker life line is one that appears chained, broken, feathery, islanded, faint or indistinct. Such a weak line denotes a delicate constitution and a tendency to run out of fuel easily. For weaker life lines, preventive health measures that boost vitality like exercising, eating right for your type, cultivating life-supporting habits and meditating to connect to our true nature are extremely important.

To sum it up, the life line is where we look at the palm to see the general level of life force, health and vitality of a person. The stronger this line is, the more curved into the palm, and the longer it is, the more energy, stamina, and fortitude is present in the life of the person. These life lines indicate a robust constitution that is blessed with the gift of reasonable health, all other things being equal.

The more the life line is short, narrowly hugging the thumb, straight, and poorly marked, the more the life energy is likely to be challenged or restricted in some way. For these people, health and cultivating vitality are a priority. It is also true that a challenged life line, and the often associated vulnerable health or health crisis that go along with such a line, can also function as an initiation into great spirituality. There is nothing like the vivid reminder of the impermanence of life to turn our hearts towards that which is eternal.

Sunday
23

Bharaṇī			28:17	
Ś 11			15:49	
Śiva			11:20	
Viṣṭi			15:49	
Bava			29:10	
Rāhu Kālam	15:41	-	16:52	
Rāhu: Libra			5:51	
Ketu: Aries			5:51	

Monday
24

Kṛttikā			Full Night	
Ś 12			18:32	
Siddha			12:17	
Bālava			18:32	
Kaulava			Full Night	
Rāhu Kālam	8:33	-	9:45	
Moon: Taurus			11:04	Christmas Eve

Tuesday
25

Kṛttikā			7:27	
Ś 13			21:18	
Sādhya			13:17	
Kaulava			7:56	
Taitila			21:18	
Rāhu Kālam	14:13	-	15:42	Christmas Day

Wednesday
26

Rohinī			10:34	
Ś 14			23:56	
Śubha			14:14	
Gara			10:38	
Vanija			23:56	
Rāhu Kālam	12:08	-	13:20	

Thursday ○
27

Mṛgaśīrṣa			13:31
Pūrṇimā			26:21
Śukla			15:03
Viṣṭi			13:11
Bava			26:21
Rāhu Kālam	13:20	-	14:32
Moon: Gemini			0:04
Mercury: Sagittarius			8:37

Friday
28

Ārdrā			16:13
K 1			28:27
Brahma			15:38
Bālava			15:26
Kaulava			28:27
Rāhu Kālam	10:58	-	12:09

Saturday
29

Punarvasu			18:35
K 2			30:12
Mahendra			15:59
Taitila			17:22
Gara			30:12
Rāhu Kālam	9:47	-	10:58
Moon: Cancer			12:02

December 2012

S	M	T	W	T	F	S
						1
2	3	4	5	6	7	8
9	10	11	12	13	14	15
16	17	18	19	20	21	22
23	24	25	26	27	28	29
30	31					

4	Mo 5	Ke JuR 6	7
3			8
Ma 2			9
Su As 1	Ra Ve Me 12	Sa 11	10

January 2013

S	M	T	W	T	F	S
		1	2	3	4	5
6	7	8	9	10	11	12
13	14	15	16	17	18	19
20	21	22	23	24	25	26
27	28	29	30	31		

Sunday

30

Puṣyā		20:37	
K 3		Full Night	
Vaidhṛti		16:04	
Vanija		18:55	
Viṣṭi		Full Night	
Rāhu Kālam	15:45	- 16:57	

Monday

31

Āśleṣā		22:15	
K 3		7:33	
Viṣkambha		15:50	
Viṣṭi		7:33	
Bava		20:05	
Rāhu Kālam	8:36	- 9:47	
Moon: Leo		22:15	

Tuesday

1

Maghā		23:27	
K 4		8:30	
Prīti		15:17	
Bālavs		8:30	
Kaulava		20:48	
Rāhu Kālam	14:35	- 15:47	New Year's Day

Wednesday

2

Pūrva Phalguṇī		24:12	
K 5		8:59	
Āyuṣman		14:23	
Taitila		8:59	
Gara		21:02	
Rāhu Kālam	12:12	- 13:24	

Thursday
3

Uttara Phalguṇī			24:28
K 6			8:58
Saubhāgya			13:05
Vanija			8:58
Viṣṭi			20:46
Rāhu Kālam	13:24	-	14:36
Moon: Virgo			6:19

Friday
4

Hasta			24:11
K 7			8:26
K 8			31:20
Śobhana			11:22
Bava			8:26
Bālava			19:57
Kaulava			31:20
Rāhu Kālam	11:01	-	12:13
Venus: Sagittarius			2:02

Saturday
5

Citrā			23:21
K 9			29:41
Atigaṇḍa			9:13
Sukarmā			30:38
Taitila			18:35
Gara			29:41
Rāhu Kālam	9:49	-	11:01
Moon: Libra			11:50

December 2012

S	M	T	W	T	F	S
						1
2	3	4	5	6	7	8
9	10	11	12	13	14	15
16	17	18	19	20	21	22
23	24	25	26	27	28	29
30	31					

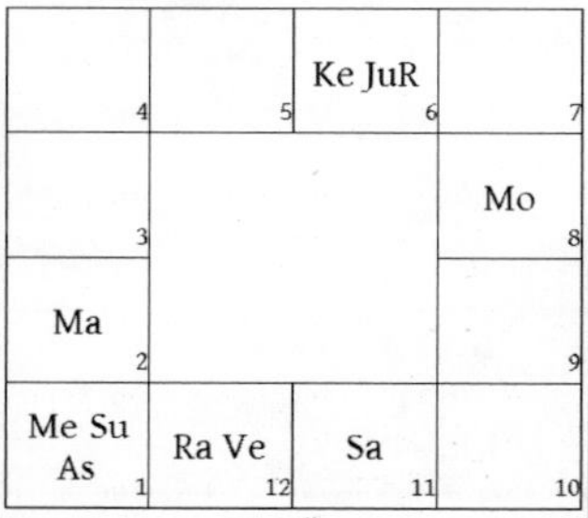

January 2013

S	M	T	W	T	F	S
		1	2	3	4	5
6	7	8	9	10	11	12
13	14	15	16	17	18	19
20	21	22	23	24	25	26
27	28	29	30	31		

Sunday

6

Svātī			22:00
K 10			27:31
Dhṛti			27:38
Vanija			16:40
Viṣṭi			27:31
Rāhu Kālam	15:50	-	17:03

Monday

7

Viśākhā			20:09
K 11			24:51
Śūla			24:14
Bava			14:14
Bālava			24:51
Rāhu Kālam	8:37	-	9:49
Moon: Scorpio			14:39

Tuesday

8

Anurādhā			17:54
K 12			21:49
Gaṇḍa			20:32
Kaulava			11:23
Taitila			21:49
Rāhu Kālam	14:40	-	15:52

Wednesday

9

Jyeṣṭhā			15:21
K 13			18:31
Vṛddhi			16:36
Viṣṭi			28:49
Gara			8:11
Vanija			18:31
Rāhu Kālam	12:15	-	13:28

Thursday
10

Mūla			12:41
K 14			15:06
Druva			12:34
Śakuni			15:06
Catuṣpada			25:24
Rāhu Kālam	13:28	-	14:41

Friday
11

Pūrvāṣāḍhā			10:02
Āmāvasyā			11:43
Vyāghāta			8:33
Harṣaṇa			28:41
Nāga			11:43
Kiṃsthughna			22:06
Rāhu Kālam	11:03	-	12:16
Moon: Capricorn			15:23

Saturday
12

Uttarāṣāḍhā			7:35
Śravaṇa			29:31
Ś 1			8:34
Ś 2			29:49
Vajra			25:08
Bava			8:34
Bālava			19:08
Kaulava			29:49
Rāhu Kālam	9:50	-	11:03

January 2013

S	M	T	W	T	F	S
		1	2	3	4	5
6	7	8	9	10	11	12
13	14	15	16	17	18	19
20	21	22	23	24	25	26
27	28	29	30	31		

4	5	Ke JuR 6	7
3			8
Ma 2			9
Ve Me Su As 1	Ra 12	Mo Sa 11	10

February 2013

S	M	T	W	T	F	S
					1	2
3	4	5	6	7	8	9
10	11	12	13	14	15	16
17	18	19	20	21	22	23
24	25	26	27	28		

Sunday
13

Dhaniṣṭhā		28:01
Ś 3		27:37
Siddhi		22:00
Taitila		16:38
Gara		27:38
Rāhu Kālam	15:52	- 17:10
Moon: Aquarius		16:41
Sun: Capricorn		17:23

Puṇya Kāla: 7:24 - 17:23

real new Year

Monday
very important to pray

14

Śatabhiṣā		27:14
Ś 4		26:10
Vyatīpāta		19:25
Vanija		14:48
Viṣṭi		26:10
Rāhu Kālam	14:35	- 15:47

Makara Saṅkrāntī • Pongal

Tuesday
" Pray "

15

Pūrva Bhādrapadā		27:16
Ś 5		25:32
Varīyān		17:29
Bava		13:44
Bālava		25:32
Rāhu Kālam	14:45	- 15:58
Moon: Pisces		21:11
Mercury: Capricorn		9:17

Wednesday
16

Uttara Bhādrapadā		28:10
Ś 6		25:47
Parigha		16:13
Kaulava		13:33
Taitila		25:47
Rāhu Kālam	12:18	- 13:31

Thursday

17

Revatī			29:52
Ś 7			26:54
Śiva			15:38
Gara			14:14
Vanija			26:54
Rāhu Kālam	13:32	-	14:46

Friday

18

Aśviṇī			Full Night
Ś 8			28:45
Siddha			15:40
Viṣṭi			15:45
Bava			28:45
Rāhu Kālam	11:04	-	12:18
Moon: Aries			5:52

Saturday

19

Aśviṇī			8:16
Ś 9			31:09
Sādhya			16:10
Balava			17:54
Kaulava			31:09
Rāhu Kālam	9:50	-	11:04

January 2013

S	M	T	W	T	F	S
		1	2	3	4	5
6	7	8	9	10	11	12
13	14	15	16	17	18	19
20	21	22	23	24	25	26
27	28	29	30	31		

4	5	Ke JuR 6	7
3			8
Ma Mo 2			9
Ve As Me Su 1	Ra 12	Sa 11	10

February 2013

S	M	T	W	T	F	S
					1	2
3	4	5	6	7	8	9
10	11	12	13	14	15	16
17	18	19	20	21	22	23
24	25	26	27	28		

Sunday

20

Bharaṇī			11:10	
Ś 10			Full Night	
Śubha			17:02	
Taitila			20:30	
Gara			Full Night	
Rāhu Kālam	16:02	-	17:17	
Moon: Taurus			17:56	

Monday

21

Kṛttikā			14:18	
Ś 10			9:52	
Śukla			18:02	
Gara			9:52	
Vanija			23:16	
Rāhu Kālam	8:35	-	9:50	Martin Luther King Jr. Day

Tuesday

22

Rohinī			17:27
Ś 11			12:38
Brahma			19:01
Viṣṭi			12:38
Bava			25:57
Rāhu Kālam	14:49	-	16:04

Wednesday

23

Mṛgaśīrṣa			20:25
Ś 12			15:13
Mahendra			19:51
Bālava			15:13
Kaulava			28:24
Rāhu Kālam	12:20	-	13:35
Moon: Gemini			6:58

Thursday

24

Ārdrā			23:02
Ś 13			17:28
Vaidhṛti			20:24
Taitila			17:28
Gara			30:26
Rāhu Kālam	13:35	-	14:51

Friday

25

Punarvasu			25:13
Ś 14			19:17
Viṣkamba			20:38
Vanija			19:17
Viṣṭi			Full Night
Rāhu Kālam	11:04	-	12:20
Moon: Cancer			18:43
Mars: Aquarius			5:02

Saturday ○

26

Puṣyā			26:58	
Pūrṇimā			20:38	
Prīti			20:31	
Viṣṭi			8:01	
Bava			20:38	
Rāhu Kālam	9:49	-	11:04	Thai Poosam

January 2013

S	M	T	W	T	F	S
		1	2	3	4	5
6	7	8	9	10	11	12
13	14	15	16	17	18	19
20	21	22	23	24	25	26
27	28	29	30	31		

3	Mo Ke 4	JuR 5	6
2			7
As Su Me Ma 1			8
Ve 12	11	Sa Ra 10	9

February 2013

S	M	T	W	T	F	S
					1	2
3	4	5	6	7	8	9
10	11	12	13	14	15	16
17	18	19	20	21	22	23
24	25	26	27	28		

Sunday

27

Āśleṣā			28:16
K 1			21:31
Āyuṣman			20:03
Bālava			9:08
Kaulava			21:31
Rāhu Kālam	16:09	-	17:25

Monday

28

Maghā			29:10
K 2			21:58
Saubhagya			19:15
Taitila			9:47
Gara			21:57
Rāhu Kālam	8:32	-	9:48
Moon: Leo			4:16
Venus: Capricorn			0:40

Tuesday

29

Pūrva Phalgunī			29:42
K 3			22:01
Śobhana			18:08
Vanija			10:02
Viṣṭi			22:01
Rāhu Kālam	14:54	-	16:10

Wednesday

30

Uttara Phalgunī			29:53
K 4			21:43
Atigaṇḍa			16:45
Bava			9:54
Bālava			21:42
Rāhu Kālam	12:21	-	13:38
Moon: Virgo			11:46

Thursday

31

Hasta		29:44
K 5		21:03
Sukarmā		15:05
Kaulava		9:25
Taitila		21:03
Rāhu Kālam	13:38	- 14:55

Friday

1

Citrā		29:15	
K 6		20:04	
Dhṛti		13:10	
Gara		8:36	
Vanija		20:04	
Rāhu Kālam	11:04	- 12:21	
Moon: Libra		17:32	
Mercury: Aquarius		20:58	Imbolc

Saturday

2

Svātī		28:26	
K 7		18:44	
Śūla		10:58	
Viṣṭi		7:26	
Bava		18:44	
Bālava		29:56	
Rāhu Kālam	9:46	- 11:04	Candlemas • Groundhog Day

January 2013

S	M	T	W	T	F	S
		1	2	3	4	5
6	7	8	9	10	11	12
13	14	15	16	17	18	19
20	21	22	23	24	25	26
27	28	29	30	31		

3	Ke 4	JuR 5	6
Ma 2			Mo 7
As Su Me 1			8
Ve 12	11	Sa Ra 10	9

February 2013

S	M	T	W	T	F	S
					1	2
3	4	5	6	7	8	9
10	11	12	13	14	15	16
17	18	19	20	21	22	23
24	25	26	27	28		

Sunday

3

Viśākhā			27:17
K 8			17:03
Gaṇḍa			8:31
Vṛddhi			29:46
Kaulava			17:03
Taitila			28:05
Rāhu Kālam	16:15	-	17:32
Moon: Scorpio			21:36

Monday

4

Anurādha			25:48
K 9			15:02
Dhruva			26:46
Gara			15:02
Vanija			25:54
Rāhu Kālam	8:28	-	9:46

Tuesday

5

Jyeṣṭhā			24:02
K 10			12:42
Vyāghāta			23:32
Viṣṭi			12:42
Bava			23:26
Rāhu Kālam	14:58	-	16:16

Wednesday

6

Mūla			22:04
K 11			10:06
Harṣaṇa			20:08
Bālava			10:07
Kaulava			20:45
Rāhu Kālam	12:22	-	13:40
Moon: Sagittarius			0:02

Thursday

7

Pūrva Āṣāḍhā		19:59
K 12		7:21
K 13		28:32
Vajra		16:38
Taitila		7:21
Gara		17:57
Vanija		28:33
Rāhu Kālam	13:41	- 14:59

Friday

8

Uttara Āṣāḍhā		17:56
K 14		25:49
Siddhi		13:08
Viṣṭi		15:09
Śakuni		25:49
Rāhu Kālam	11:03	- 12:22
Moon: Capricorn		1:28

Saturday ●

9

Śravaṇa		16:03
Āmāvasyā		23:20
Vyatīpāta		9:46
Varīyān		30:38
Catuṣpada		12:32
Nāga		23:20
Rāhu Kālam	9:43	- 11:03

February 2013

S	M	T	W	T	F	S
					1	2
3	4	5	6	7	8	9
10	11	12	13	14	15	16
17	18	19	20	21	22	23
24	25	26	27	28		

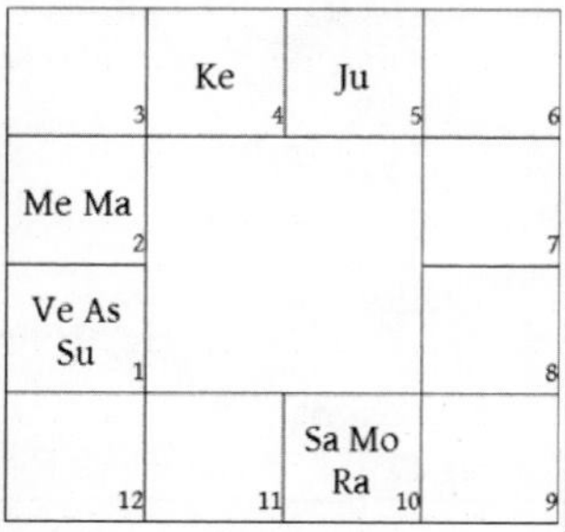

March 2013

S	M	T	W	T	F	S
					1	2
3	4	5	6	7	8	9
10	11	12	13	14	15	16
17	18	19	20	21	22	23
24	25	26	27	28		

Sunday

10

Dhaniṣṭhā			14:31	
Ś 1			21:14	
Parigha			27:52	
Kiṃstughna			10:13	
Bava			21:14	
Rāhu Kālam	16:21	-	17:40	
Moon: Aquarius			3:14	Chinese New Year: Year of the Snake

Monday

11

Śatabhiṣā			13:29	
Ś 2			19:43	
Śiva			25:34	
Bālava			8:24	
Kaulava			19:43	
Rāhu Kālam	8:22	-	9:42	

Tuesday

12

Pūrva Bhādrapadā			13:07	
Ś 3			18:52	
Siddha			23:51	
Taitila			7:12	
Gara			18:52	
Vanija			30:45	
Rāhu Kālam	15:02	-	16:22	
Moon: Pisces			7:08	Mardi Gras
Sun: Aquarius			6:24	Puṇya Kāla: 7:02 - 12:22

Wednesday

13

Uttara Bhādrapadā			13:29	
Ś 4			18:49	
Sādhya			22:45	
Viṣṭi			18:49	
Bava			Full Night	
Rāhu Kālam	12:22	-	13:42	Ash Wednesday

Thursday

14

Revatī		14:38	
Ś 5		19:35	
Śubha		22:17	
Bava		7:06	
Bālava		19:35	
Rāhu Kālam	13:43	- 15:03	
Moon: Aries		14:38	Vasant Pañcamī • Valentine's Day

Friday

15

Aśvinī		16:32
Ś 6		21:06
Śukla		22:23
Kaulava		8:15
Taitila		21:06
Rāhu Kālam	11:01	- 12:22

Saturday

16

Bharaṇī		19:04
Ś 7		23:15
Brahma		22:57
Gara		10:07
Vanija		23:16
Rāhu Kālam	9:39	- 11:00

February 2013

S	M	T	W	T	F	S
					1	2
3	4	5	6	7	8	9
10	11	12	13	14	15	16
17	18	19	20	21	22	23
24	25	26	27	28		

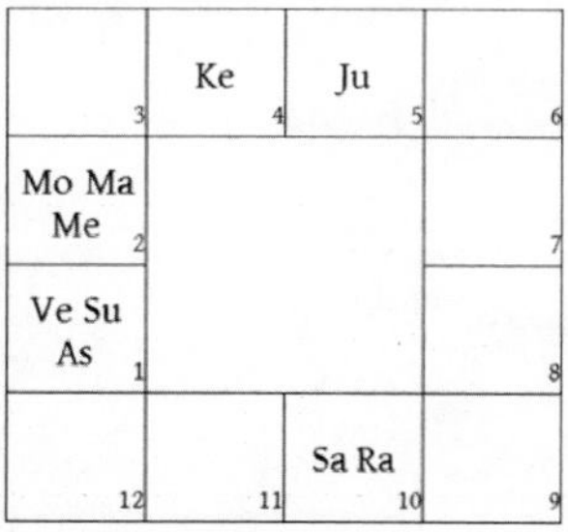

March 2013

S	M	T	W	T	F	S
					1	2
3	4	5	6	7	8	9
10	11	12	13	14	15	16
17	18	19	20	21	22	23
24	25	26	27	28		

Sunday

17

Kṛttikā		22:01	
Ś 8		25:49	
Mahendra		23:49	
Viṣṭi		12:30	
Bava		25:49	
Rāhu Kālam	16:26 -	17:48	
Moon: Taurus		1:47	

Monday

18

Rohinī		25:08	
Ś 9		28:30	
Vaidhṛti		24:48	
Bālava		15:10	
Kaulava		28:30	
Rāhu Kālam	8:16 -	9:38	President's Day

Tuesday

19

Mṛgaśīrṣa		28:10	
Ś 10		Full Night	
Viṣkhamba		25:43	
Taitila		17:49	
Gara		Full Night	
Rāhu Kālam	15:06 -	16:28	
Moon: Gemini		14:41	

Wednesday

20

Ārdrā		Full Night	
Ś 10		7:04	
Prīti		26:24	
Gara		7:04	
Vanija		20:13	
Rāhu Kālam	12:21 -	13:44	
Venus: Aquarius		23:42	

Thursday

21

Ārdrā			6:52
Ś 11			9:15
Āyuṣman			26:43
Viṣṭi			9:15
Bava			22:10
Rāhu Kālam	13:44	-	15:07

Friday

22

Punarvasu			9:06	
Ś 12			10:56	
Saubhagya			26:36	
Bālava			10:56	
Kaulava			23:33	
Rāhu Kālam	10:58	-	12:21	
Moon: Cancer			2:35	Purim Starts (sunset)

Saturday

23

Pūṣya			10:45	
Ś 13			12:01	
Śobhana			26:01	
Taitila			12:01	
Gara			24:20	
Rāhu Kālam	9:34	-	10:58	Purim Ends (sunset)

February 2013

S	M	T	W	T	F	S
					1	2
3	4	5	6	7	8	9
10	11	12	13	14	15	16
17	18	19	20	21	22	23
24	25	26	27	28		

2	Ke 3	Mo Ju 4	5
Su As Ma Me 1			6
Ve 12			7
11	10	Sa Ra 9	8

March 2013

S	M	T	W	T	F	S
					1	2
3	4	5	6	7	8	9
10	11	12	13	14	15	16
17	18	19	20	21	22	23
24	25	26	27	28		

Sunday

24

Āśleṣā			11:50
Ś 14			12:30
Atigaṇḍa			25:00
Vanija			12:30
Viṣṭi			24:32
Rāhu Kālam	16:32	-	17:55
Moon: Leo			11:50

Monday ○

25

Maghā			12:23
Pūrṇimā			12:26
Sukarmā			23:35
Bava			12:26
Bālava			24:12
Rāhu Kālam	8:09	-	9:33

Tuesday

26

Pūrva Phalgunī			12:28
K 1			11:53
Dhṛti			21:49
Kaulava			11:53
Taitila			23:27
Rāhu Kālam	15:09	-	16:33
Moon: Virgo			18:25

Wednesday

27

Uttara Phalgunī			12:10
K 2			10:57
Śūla			19:47
Gara			10:57
Vanija			22:22
Rāhu Kālam	12:21	-	13:45

Thursday

28

Hasta			11:35
K 3			9:43
Gaṇḍa			17:33
Viṣṭi			9:43
Bava			21:00
Rāhu Kālam	13:45	-	15:10
Moon: Libra			23:12

Friday

1

Citrā			10:47
K 4			8:14
K 5			30:35
Vṛddhi			15:08
Bālava			8:14
Kaualava			19:26
Taitila			30:35
Rāhu Kālam	10:55	-	12:20

Saturday

2

Svāti			9:48
K 6			28:47
Dhruva			12:35
Gara			17:42
Vanija			28:47
Rāhu Kālam	9:29	-	10:54

February 2013

S	M	T	W	T	F	S
					1	2
3	4	5	6	7	8	9
10	11	12	13	14	15	16
17	18	19	20	21	22	23
24	25	26	27	28		

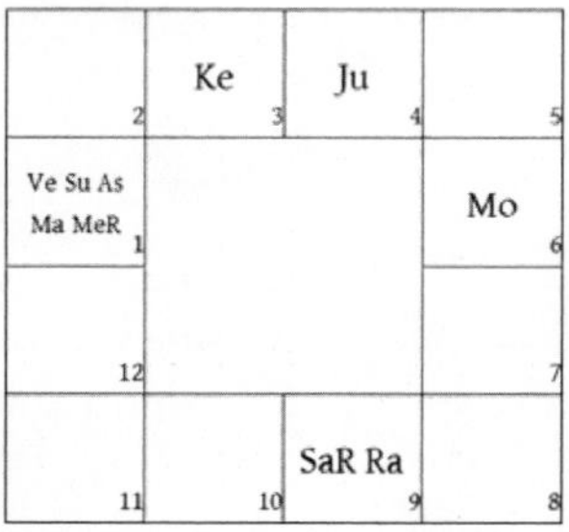

March 2013

S	M	T	W	T	F	S
					1	2
3	4	5	6	7	8	9
10	11	12	13	14	15	16
17	18	19	20	21	22	23
24	25	26	27	28		

Sunday

3

Viśākhā			8:41
K 7			26:52
Vyāghāta			9:55
Viṣṭi			15:51
Bava			26:52
Rāhu Kālam	16:37	-	18:02
Moon: Scorpio			2:58

Monday

4

Anurādha			7:27
Jyeṣṭhā			30:07
K 8			24:51
Harṣaṇa			7:10
Vajra			28:20
Bālava			13:53
Kaualava			24:51
Rāhu Kālam	8:01	-	9:27
Mars: Pisces			7:09

Tuesday

5

Mūla			28:43
K 9			22:45
Siddhi			25:27
Taitila			11:49
Gara			22:45
Rāhu Kālam	15:12	-	16:38
Moon: Sagittarius			6:07

Wednesday

6

Pūrva Āṣāḍhā			27:17
K 10			20:36
Vyatīpāta			22:32
Vanija			9:41
Viṣṭi			20:37
Rāhu Kālam	12:19	-	13:36

Thursday

7

Uttara Āṣāḍhā			25:52
K 11			18:28
Varīyān			19:37
Bava			7:32
Bālava			18:28
Kaulava			29:26
Rāhu Kālam	13:45	-	15:12
Moon: Capricorn			8:55

Friday

8

Śravaṇa			24:35
K 12			16:26
Parigha			16:47
Taitila			16:26
Gara			27:28
Rāhu Kālam	10:51	-	12:18

Saturday

9

Dhaniṣṭhā			23:32	
K 13			14:34	
Śiva			14:06	
Vanija			14:34	
Viṣṭi			25:44	
Rāhu Kālam	9:23	-	10:51	
Moon: Aquarius			12:01	Mahā Śiva Rātrī

March 2013

S	M	T	W	T	F	S
					1	2
3	4	5	6	7	8	9
10	11	12	13	14	15	16
17	18	19	20	21	22	23
24	25	26	27	28		

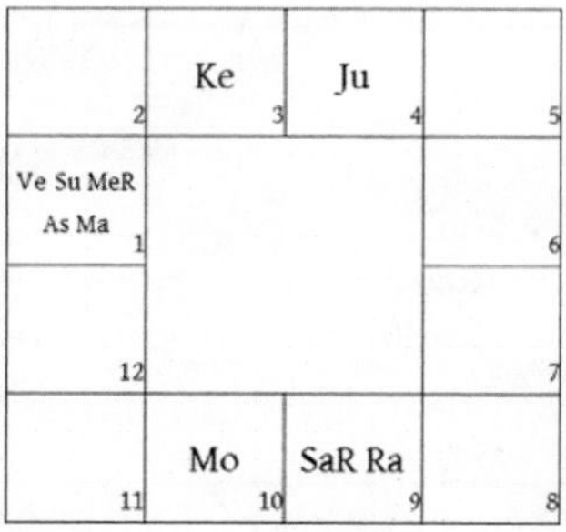

April 2013

S	M	T	W	T	F	S
	1	2	3	4	5	6
7	8	9	10	11	12	13
14	15	16	17	18	19	20
21	22	23	24	25	26	27
28	29	30				

Sunday

10

Śatabhiṣā		23:48	
K 14		14:00	
Siddha		12:40	
Śakuni		14:00	
Catuṣpada		25:22	
Rāhu Kālam	17:41 -	19:09	Daylight Savings Starts

Monday

11

Pūrva Bhādrapada		23:32
Āmāvasyā		12:51
Sādhya		10:33
Nāgava		12:51
Kiṃstughna		24:27
Rāhu Kālam	8:53 -	10:21
Moon: Pisces		17:33

Tuesday

12

Uttara Bhādrapadā		23:50
Ś 1		12:13
Subha		8:50
Bava		12:13
Bālava		24:08
Rāhu Kālam	16:14 -	17:43

Wednesday

13

Revatī		24:46
Ś 2		12:13
Śukla		7:37
Brahma		30:54
Kaulava		12:13
Taitila		24:28
Rāhu Kālam	13:17 -	14:46

Thursday

14

Aśviṇī		26:22	
Ś 3		12:53	
Mahendra		30:43	
Gara		12:53	
Vanija		25:29	
Rāhu Kālam	14:46 -	16:15	
Moon: Aries		0:46	
Sun: Pisces		4:21	Puṇya Kāla: 7:21 - 13:17

Friday

15

Bharaṇī		28:35
Ś 4		14:14
Vaidhṛti		31:01
Viṣṭi		14:14
Bava		27:08
Rāhu Kālam	11:47 -	13:16

Saturday

16

Kṛttikā		Full Night
Ś 5		16:10
Viṣkhambha		Full Night
Bālava		16:10
Kaulava		29:19
Rāhu Kālam	10:17 -	11:47
Moon: Taurus		11:13

March 2013

S	M	T	W	T	F	S
					1	2
3	4	5	6	7	8	9
10	11	12	13	14	15	16
17	18	19	20	21	22	23
24	25	26	27	28		

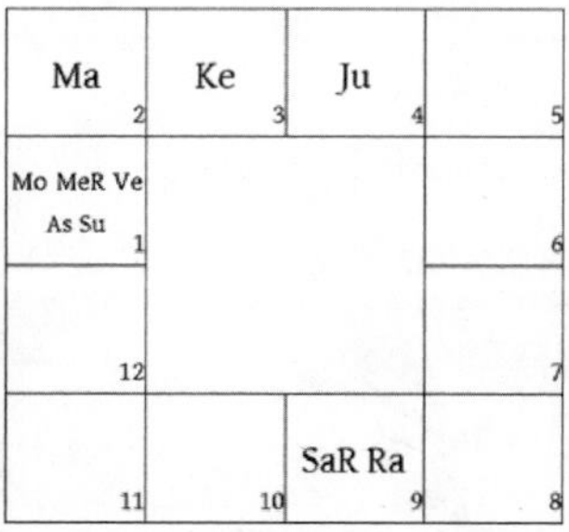

April 2013

S	M	T	W	T	F	S
	1	2	3	4	5	6
7	8	9	10	11	12	13
14	15	16	17	18	19	20
21	22	23	24	25	26	27
28	29	30				

Sunday

17

Kṛttikā			7:17	
Ś 6			18:33	
Viṣkhambha			7:41	
Taitila			18:33	
Gara			Full Night	
Rāhu Kālam	17:46	-	19:16	
Venus: Pisces			1:28	St. Patrick's Day

Monday

18

Rohiṇī			10:17	
Ś 7			21:09	
Prīti			8:36	
Gara			7:50	
Vanija			21:08	
Rāhu Kālam	8:45	-	10:15	
Moon: Gemini			23:49	

Tuesday

19

Mṛgaśīrṣa			13:21	
Ś 8			23:41	
Āyuṣman			9:35	
Viṣṭi			10:26	
Bava			23:41	
Rāhu Kālam	16:14	-	17:47	

Wednesday

20

Ārdrā			16:13	
Ś 9			25:56	
Saubhāgya			10:26	
Bālava			12:52	
Kaulava			25:56	
Rāhu Kālam	13:15	-	14:46	Ostara • Spring Equinox 4:02

Thursday

21

Punarvasu		18:41
Ś 10		27:40
Śobhana		10:59
Taitila		14:52
Gara		27:40
Rāhu Kālam	14:46	- 16:17
Moon: Cancer		12:07

Friday

22

Puṣyā		20:34
Ś 11		28:46
Atigaṇḍa		11:07
Vanija		16:18
Viṣṭi		28:45
Rāhu Kālam	11:43	- 13:15

Saturday

23

Āśleṣā		21:46
Ś 12		29:09
Sukarmā		10:44
Bava		17:02
Bālava		29:09
Rāhu Kālam	10:11	- 11:42
Moon: Leo		21:46

March 2013

S	M	T	W	T	F	S
					1	2
3	4	5	6	7	8	9
10	11	12	13	14	15	16
17	18	19	20	21	22	23
24	25	26	27	28		

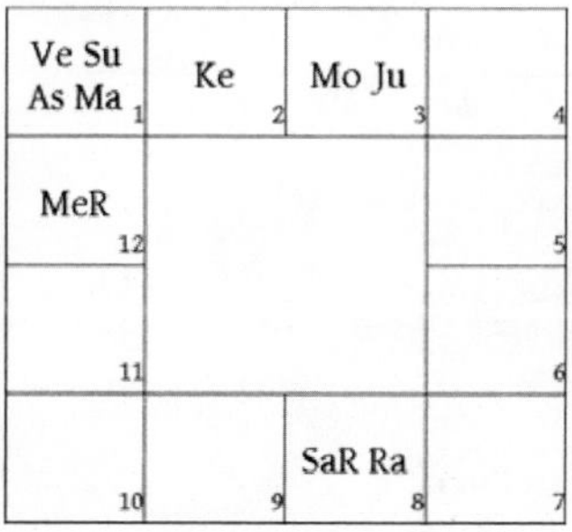

April 2013

S	M	T	W	T	F	S
	1	2	3	4	5	6
7	8	9	10	11	12	13
14	15	16	17	18	19	20
21	22	23	24	25	26	27
28	29	30				

Sunday

24

Maghā		22:18	
Ś 13		28:50	
Dhṛti		9:48	
Kaulava		17:04	
Taitila		28:50	
Rāhu Kālam	17:50 -	19:22	Palm Sunday

Monday

25

Pūrva Phalgunī		22:12	
Ś 14		27:54	
Śūla		8:21	
Gaṇḍa		30:25	
Gara		16:27	
Vanija		27:54	
Rāhu Kālam	8:36 -	10:09	Passover Begins

Tuesday ○

26

Uttara Phalgunī		21:33	
Pūrṇimā		26:27	
Vṛddhi		28:04	
Viṣṭi		15:14	
Bava		26:27	
Rāhu Kālam	16:19 -	17:51	Holī • Lakṣmī Jayantī

Wednesday

27

Hasta		20:28	
K 1		24:35	
Dhruva		25:23	
Bālava		13:33	
Kaulava		24:35	
Rāhu Kālam	13:13 -	14:46	

Thursday

28

Citrā			19:05
K 2			22:25
Vyāghāta			22:29
Taitila			11:31
Gara			22:25
Rāhu Kālam	14:46	-	16:19
Moon: Libra			7:48

Friday

29

Svāti			17:30
K 3			20:04
Harṣaṇa			19:26
Vanija			9:15
Viṣṭi			20:04
Bava			30:51
Rāhu Kālam	11:39	-	13:12

Good Friday

Saturday

30

Viśākhā			15:49
K 4			17:38
Vajra			16:19
Bālava			17:38
Kaulava			28:25
Rāhu Kālam	10:05	-	11:38
Moon: Scorpio			10:15

March 2013

S	M	T	W	T	F	S
					1	2
3	4	5	6	7	8	9
10	11	12	13	14	15	16
17	18	19	20	21	22	23
24	25	26	27	28		

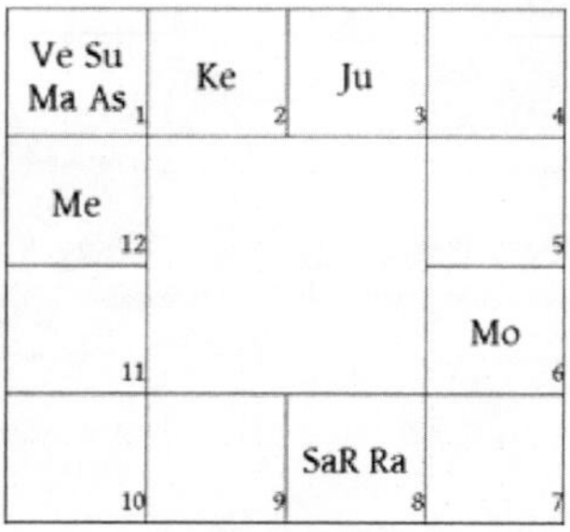

April 2013

S	M	T	W	T	F	S
	1	2	3	4	5	6
7	8	9	10	11	12	13
14	15	16	17	18	19	20
21	22	23	24	25	26	27
28	29	30				

Chapter Three

~

SPRING

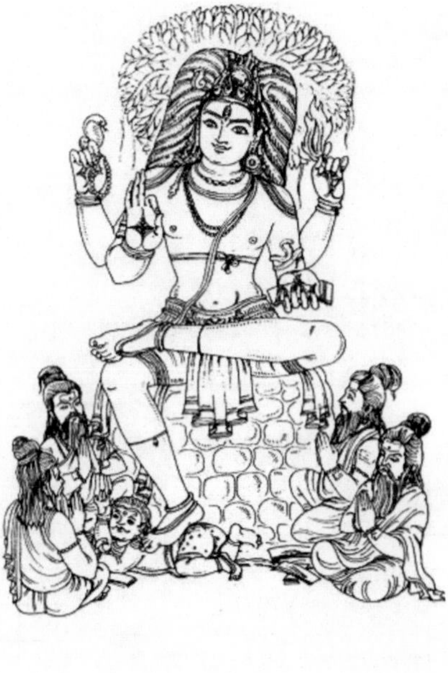

Dakṣiṇāmūrti Stotram

Part 2

Verse 1

Viśvaṃ darpaṇadṛśyamānanagarītulyaṃ nijāntargataṃ
Paśyannātmani māyayā bahirivodbhūtaṃ yathā nidrayā |
Yaḥ sākṣāt kurute prabodha samaye svātmānam evā dvayaṃ
Tasmai śrīgurumūrtaye nama idaṃ śrīdakṣiṇāmūrtaye ||

Viśvaṁ - the entire manifest universe; Darpaṇa – a mirror; Dṛśya – seen; Māna – the space of; Nagarī – city; Tulyaṁ - like, equal to; Nija – the Self; Antargataṁ - existing within; Paśyann – seeing; Ātmāni – in one's Self; Māyayā – by illusion; Bahi – outside; Iva – as though; .Ūdbhūtaṁ - appears; Yathā – just as; Nidrayā – like in a dream

Yaḥ - he who; Sākṣāt – is seen; Kurute – made; Prabodha – awakening; Samaye – at the time of; Svātmānam – his own Self; Eva – one; Advayaṁ - without a second; Tasmai – to him; Śrīguru – respected teacher; Mūrtaye – in the form; Nama – salutations; Idaṁ - this; Śrīdakṣiṇamūrtaye – respected One facing South

In an illusory dream everything is perceived of as being mirrored outside of oneself. In reality, the space of this entire creation exists entirely within one's own Self. My deepest salutations to my respected teacher in the form of Dakṣiṇāmūrti.

Verse 2

Bījasya antariva aṅkuro jagadidaṃ prāṅnirvikalpaṁ punaḥ
Māyākalpitadeśakālakalanāvaicitryacitrīkṛtam |
Māyāvīva vijṛmbhayatyapi mahāyogīva yaḥ svecchayā
tasmai śrīgurumūrtaye nama idaṃ śrīdakṣiṇāmūrtaye ||

Bījasya – a seed's; Antar – inside; Iva – like; Aṅkuraḥ - a sprout; Jagad – universe; Idam – this; Prā – before, at the beginning; Nirvikalpam – unmanifest; Punaḥ - after; Māyā – illusion; Kalpita – projected; Deśa –

space; Kāla – time; Kalanā – causing; Vaicitrya – certainly manifest; Citrī – manifest; Kṛtaṁ - made

Māyāvī – a magician; Iva – just like; Vijṛmbhayati – projects; Api – even; Mahā – great; Yogi – master; Iva – like; Yaḥ - he who; Sveccha – [sva + iccha] – his own desire; Tasmai...

Just like a sprout is hidden inside of a seed, this whole Universe was in a similar primordial state before it had manifested. Certainly, just like a magician portrays illusion as reality, Māyā, through the medium of time and space, portrays this Universe as real. That great Yogi, Dakṣiṇāmūrti, by his will sees the whole of Creation as both within and outside of himself. My deepest salutations to my respected teacher in the form of Dakṣiṇāmūrti.

Verse 3

Yasyaiva sphuraṇaṃ sadātmakam asat kalpārthagaṃ bhāsate
Sākṣāt tattvamas īti vedavacasā yo bodhayat yāśritān |
Yat sākṣāt karaṇād bhavenna punara avṛttir bhavām bhonidhau
Tasmai śrīgurumūrtaye nama idaṃ śrīdakṣiṇāmūrtaye ||

Yasya – for whom; Eva – indeed; Sphuraṇaṁ - consciousness; Sat – truth; Ātmākam – the Self; Asat – untruth; Kalpa – like; Arthagaṁ - all of creation; Bhāsate – shines; Sākṣāt – in front of; Tattvamasī – "That, you are!"; Iti – sayeth; Veda – the scriptures; Vacasā – by the words of; Yaḥ - he who; Bodhayati – causes to know; Āśritān – those sitting in front of

Yat – of whom; Sākṣāt – in front of; Karaṇa – means of knowledge; Adbhavenna – is not; Punara – again; Avṛttiḥ - return; Bhava – becoming; Ambhas – heavens; Onidau – container; Tasmai...

Dakṣiṇāmūrti, understanding both the untruth which manifests as duality as well as the truth that shines as the Self, through the medium of the great affirmation which is said by the holy scriptures – "*Thou art that!*" – imparts the knowledge of the Self to the students sitting in front of him. Through this knowledge, there is no return again to the world of becoming. My deepest salutations to my respected teacher in the form of Dakṣiṇāmūrti.

Verse 4

Nānā chidra ghaṭo dara sthita mahā dīpa prabhā bhāsvaraṁ
Jñānaṃ yasya tu cakṣurādi karaṇad vārā bahiḥ spandate |
Jānāmīti tameva bhāntam anubhātye tat samaṣtaṃ jagat
Tasmai śrīgurumūrtaye nama idaṃ śrīdakṣiṇāmūrtaye ||

Nana – many, various; Chidra – whole, puncture; Ghaṭa – pot; Udara – inside; Sthita – staying, abiding, place; Mahā – great; Dīpa – lamp; Prabhā – light; Bhāsvaraṁ - shinning; Jñānaṁ - knowledge; Yasya – whose; Tu – but; Cakṣur – the eyes; Ādi – along with the rest of the senses; Karaṇa – cause; Dvārā – through; Bahiḥ - appearing to be outside; Spandate – shinning

Jānāmi – I know; Iti – thus; Tameva – verily, that only; Bhāntam – that which is illumined; Anubhāti – shines after; Etat – this; Samastaṁ - whole; Jagat – world; Tasmai...

The Self within, when directed outside through the various senses, is like a water pot with many holes in it. Verily, I know that Self to be like a great lamp abiding within that pot because it causes all things to function. My deepest salutations to my respected teacher in the form of Dakṣiṇāmūrti.

Verse 5

Dehaṃ prāṇamap īndriyāṇyapi calāṃ buddhiṃ ca śūnyaṃ viduḥ
Śrī bāla andhajaḍo pamāstv aham iti bhrāntā bhṛśaṃ vādinaḥ |
Māyā śaktivilāsa kalpita mahāvyāmoha saṃhāriṇe
Tasmai śrīgurumūrtaye nama idaṃ śrīdakṣiṇāmūrtaye ||

Dehaṁ - body; Prāṇam – vital force; Api – also; Indriyāṇi – sense organs; Api – also; Calāṁ - moving; Buddhiṁ - intellect; Ca – and; Śūnyaṁ - void, zero; Viduḥ - intellect; Śrī – woman; Bāla – child; Andha – blind person; Jaḍa –inert, not conscious, possessed by spirits; Upamās – like; Tvahaṁ – I am; Iti – verily; Brāntā – someone who is wandering, lost, wondering in circles, confused, perplexed, holding an erroneous position; Bhṛśaṁ - extremely; Vādinaḥ – someone who has a philosophical position

Māyā – of illusion; Śakti – power; Vilāsa – sport, play; Kalpita – projected, created by; Mahā – great; Vyāmoha – delusion, misconception; Saṁhāriṇe – from saṁhārin, a destroyer, one who completely destroys; Tasmai...

These self-proclaimed philosophers are extremely confused, perplexed and immature, similar to a child, blind person, or someone possessed by spirits. They, as if wandering in circles with a wavering intellect, think the body with its vital energy, senses, etc, to be the Self. To He who completely destroys these erroneous misconceptions which are projected by the play of the power of the Illusion, to my respected teacher in the form of Dakṣiṇāmūrti, salutations.

To be continued...

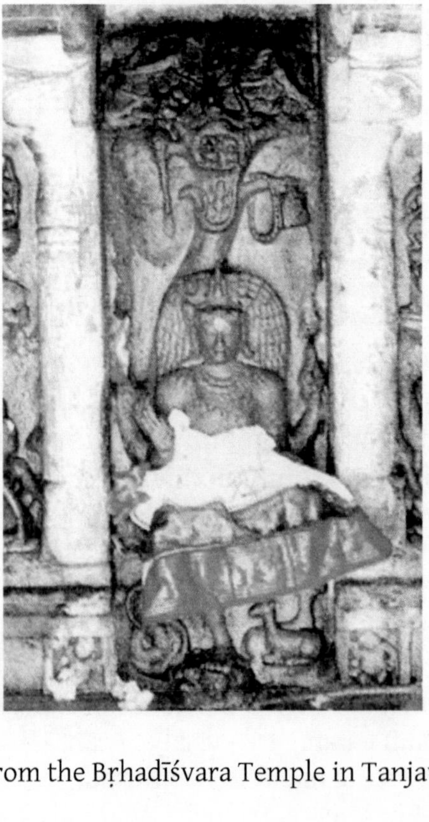

Dakṣiṇāmūrti from the Bṛhadīśvara Temple in Tanjavur, Tamiḷ Nadu

Hasta Sāmudrika Śāstra
~
The Water Hand

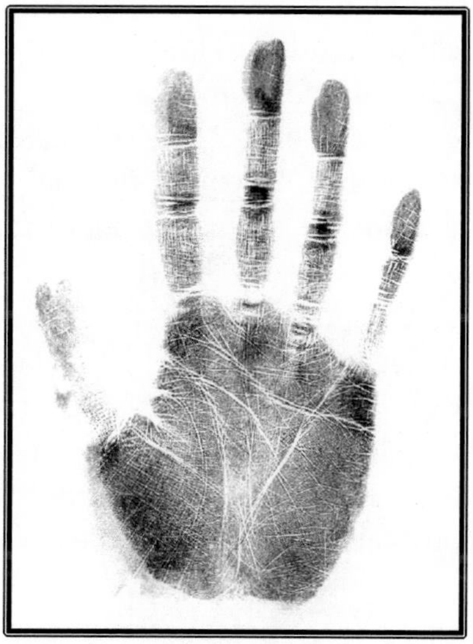

Spring arrives, melting the mountain snows and ice into water. This cool water flows deeply and nourishes the lands. Just as water permeates and nourishes our world, those with water hands are magnanimous and thoughtful towards others. The water-hand type accommodates, adapts, and is considerate and supportive to those around them in the same way that water takes its shape from what contains it. Known as the sensitive and intuitive type, water-handed people are generally refined, spiritual, and idealistic. More than any other hand type, they are able to access deep emotions and experience life's currents profoundly. This hand type is more common among women than men and the most infrequent of the hand types in general.

The Palm

Typical water hands have narrow, rectangular palms. Often the whole hand, including the palm, looks like it has been stretched out from the base of the hand to the fingers. These palms are also very pliable and flexible. Narrow palms are associated with imagination, subjectivity, instability, and uncertainty. The elongated palm forms the foundation for the water-hand type's strong emotionality. Water hands share rectangular palms in common with fire hands, just as both types of hands can be said to be emotional. But the difference between these two types is that the fire-handed person will tend to direct their emotions outward towards life, always alive, moving, enthusiastic, and curious, while the water-handed emotions are more protected and internal. A natural introspection sometimes leads the water-handed type to escape from the world into a private inner reality.

The Fingers

Water hands have the longest fingers of all the hand types, and the fingers are often delicate and very flexible, like those of some fashion models. This flexibility reflects the adaptability inherent in the water element. Just as water spreads and fills any space, water-hand people are empathic, compassionate, and kind. They are able to truly sense what other people are experiencing emotionally and their deep need for peace makes them reach out and support those around them so that all may be in balance. The evolutionary journey for water-handed people therefore includes a lifelong dance of learning how to establish appropriate boundaries and not over-extending themselves. Their need for external harmony, coupled with their versatility can often lead them to compromise their own needs for the sake of others. Learning to stay centered helps those with water hands maintain useful boundaries and avoid excessive self-sacrifice.

Skin texture

The water hand is the most refined of all the hand types. The skin is smooth and often appears shiny and satiny, even from a distance. Refined skin mirrors a refined view of life.

Those with water hands are often so idealistic and imaginative that sometimes it is hard for them to stay connected to the objective world; they are dreamers who prefer to 'feel' things instead of 'think' about them. Because water types see things more deeply than others, it is not always easy for them to articulate their experiences simply and precisely. They often just hope that others will sense what they are feeling and act accordingly. Sometimes this leads to others perceiving the person as moody.

Lines

The palm of the water type is covered with a great number of fine lines, with the principal lines standing out from the rest. The lines are usually thin, forming a shallow, web-like, tangled mass. You will see many vertical lines and lots of crisscrossing.

The water hand generally displays the greatest number of lines among the hand types. A palm so full of lines reflects how profoundly the individual's environment affects them. The things that happen around them leave traces on their inner being. This helps explain why the water-handed person is the most prone to psychosomatic disorders, fear, anxiety, and digestive complaints that have an origin in the emotional realm. They naturally have a need for lots of sleep, and a calm and peaceful environment is essential to their emotional balance and stability. Water-handed people must be careful not to push themselves beyond what their bodies are capable of.

Fingerprints

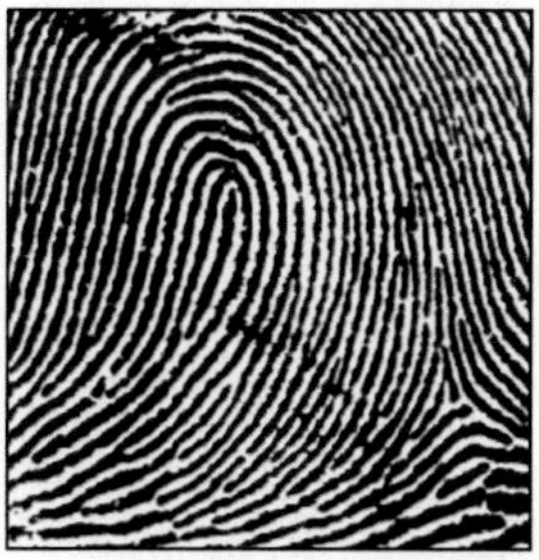

The fingerprint pattern most associated with the water hand is the loop. Loops flow in and out of the top part of the digit from one side and never turn into a whorl or closed shape. A person whose fingerprints are mainly loops tends to be easy-going and fit in well with others. The loop-dominant water-hand type is quiet and receptive, and gravitates towards situations that enable the expression of their innate sensitivity to people and beauty.

A water-handed person's natural inspiration and gentleness spontaneously arises from an understanding of life as flexible and changeable. In its most subtle form, this hand type's capacity for inner reflection becomes the seeker's impulse towards the divine.

Hasta Sāmudrika Śāstra

~

The Head Line

Head Line

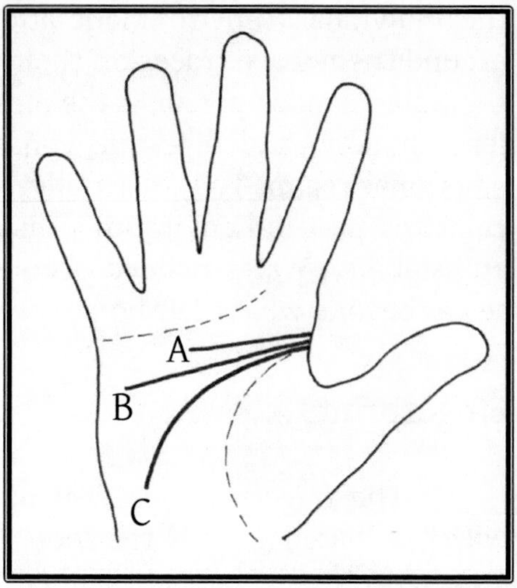

The Head Line is one of the primary lines in the human hand, and is found on every hand with no exception. It is the second horizontal line at the top of the palm. It begins on the thumb side of the hand and travels across the palm towards the little finger side. This line exhibits great variety in length, clarity, shape and position. In the diagram to the right, line *A* represents an average, straight line; line *B* shows a long, straight line and line *C* shows a long, curved line.

The head line is known as mātṛ rekhā in sanskrit. While 'rekhā' means 'line', 'mātṛ' means 'the measurer'. Indeed, this line gives lots of information about how a person measures their world and how they make sense of their environment. Everybody measures their world through the five senses, enabled by our minds, yet we all do so differently. By careful analysis of the head line we gain insight into a person's thought patterns, their capacities and their creativity. The head line reveals details about how we think and our quality of mind. It also reveals to what extent we are original and innovative in our thoughts, how much we like to dream up new things, or how much we like to stick to what is known.

The character traits revealed by the head line are valuable because we want to accurately evaluate our talents, and then find a field in which to apply them. Because we measure our world through our thoughts, certain ways of thinking are better suited for different activities. For example, a psychologist has the talent for slower, more detailed thinking than an air traffic control operator, who instead we expect to be a decisive and quick thinker.

Length

The length of the head line is directly related to how long or how quickly a person assesses their world. It reveals how elaborate or simple a person's thinking is. We have different ways of processing information, and neither is better than the other. Just as with the example of the psychologist and the air traffic controller above, we appreciate that different ways of thinking are better suited for specific situations.

An average head line is one that ends approximately under the middle of the ring finger. That means that a head line that approaches the side of the hand under the little finger is long. A head line that ends in the middle of the palm is short.

Long head lines indicate the capacity for detailed, complex thinking. These lines are found on the hands of those that are able to consider many details when thinking about something, giving them the ability for more intricate thoughts. For example, long head lines love to analyze the world, discovering more and more details about it as they go along. They enjoy problem-solving and puzzles, and generally thinking things through deeply. The downside to a long headline occurs when over-thinking or over-analyzing a situation can make decision-making difficult (analysis leads to paralysis).

Short head lines, instead, reflect the ability to be decisive and quickly assess a situation. A short head line may be found, for example, on the hand of an engineer who is capable of linear, practical, clear and simple thinking. A common palmistry misconception is that short head lines correspond with short intelligence, but this is not found to be true in experience. What is true is that, given a complex problem, a person with a short head line is less inclined to think about it for a long time. Their strategy is to try something, see if it works, and if it does not work to try something else. Someone with a long head line, on the other hand, will be more likely to think deeply about a solution and its implications before trying it.

Path

The straighter the head line, the more pragmatic the thinking process. Straight head lines are analytical, efficient, logical, practical and think of things in terms of how useful they are. These head lines are attracted to mathematics, science, technology and business. The curved headline, in contrast, is associated with creativity and imagination. The more curved a head line, the greater the imagination is likely to be and the person will enjoy doing things in new ways.

Origin

A head line that is joined at its origin with the life line is the most common and suggests a certain caution but also a reasonable and pleasant character, all other things being equal. Less frequent is the head line that is not connected to the life line and seems to float above it. This is a sign of somebody who is unique in their way of thinking and values independence in their career and their environment. The greater the gap between the life and head lines, the more spontaneity, boldness, and optimism about life.

Simian Line

There is one variation of the headline that is worth mentioning and this is when the head line and the heart line merge into one clear line that cuts horizontally all the way across the palm. This is also known as a Simian line. For most people, what one thinks (head line) and what one feels (heart line) are different things, but for the Simian line these channels converge into one and what results is laser-beam intensity. This intensity can manifest as a bold personality and an ability to persevere no matter what. In fact, the Sanskrit name for such a line is 'ākrama rekhā', whose meanings include 'attaining, approaching, obtaining and overcoming'. In an otherwise stable hand, an ākrama rekhā gives the ability to accomplish a lot through focus, leadership, and organizational capacity. Many successful people have such a line, including many wise spiritual teachers, for whom the integration of heart and mind takes them one step closer to the full integration of being with our true, infinite nature that is the hallmark of an authentic spiritual path. In a less stable hand, this line can indicate a tremendous quantity of internal stress. For those with a Simian line that are learning to manage the associated intensity, the most productive avenues of expression are through creativity and the arts, and through knowing oneself deeply (meditation, spiritual questing).

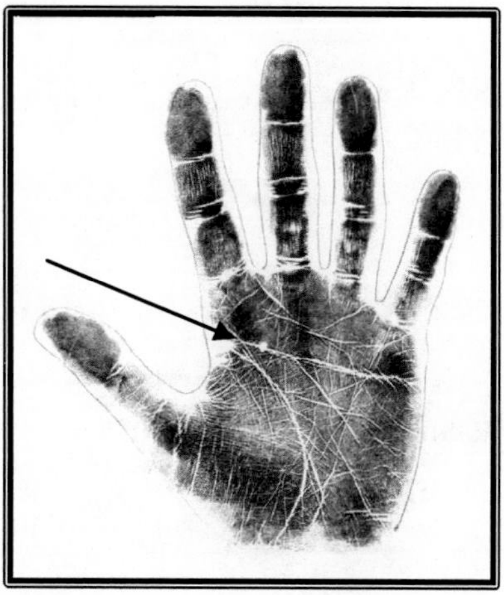

Sunday

31

Anurādhā			14:09	
K 5			15:13	
Siddhi			13:12	
Taitila			15:13	
Gara			26:02	
Rāhu Kālam	17:55	-	19:29	Easter

Monday

1

Jyeṣṭhā			12:32	
K 6			12:52	
Vyatīpāta			10:09	
Vanija			12:52	
Viṣṭi			23:44	
Rāhu Kālam	8:28	-	10:02	
Moon: Sagittarius			12:32	April Fool's Day

Tuesday

2

Mūla			11:03	
K 7			10:39	
Varīyān			7:11	
Parigha			28:22	
Bava			10:39	
Bālava			21:36	
Rāhu Kālam	16:21	-	17:56	Passover Finishes

Wednesday

3

Pūrvāṣāḍhā			9:45	
K 8			8:36	
K 9			30:46	
Śiva			25:42	
Kaulava			8:36	
Taitila			19:39	
Gara			30:46	
Rāhu Kālam	13:11	-	14:46	
Moon: Capricorn			15:27	

Thursday

4

Uttarāṣāḍhā		8:39
K 10		29:10
Siddha		23:14
Vanija		17:56
Viṣṭi		29:10
Rāhu Kālam	14:46	- 16:21

Friday

5

Śravaṇa		7:48
K 11		27:52
Sādhya		21:00
Bava		16:29
Bālava		27:52
Rāhu Kālam	11:35	- 13:10
Moon: Aquarius		19:29

Saturday

6

Dhaniṣṭhā		7:15
K 12		26:54
Śubha		19:01
Kaulava		15:21
Taitila		26:54
Rāhu Kālam	9:58	- 11:34

March 2013

S	M	T	W	T	F	S
					1	2
3	4	5	6	7	8	9
10	11	12	13	14	15	16
17	18	19	20	21	22	23
24	25	26	27	28		

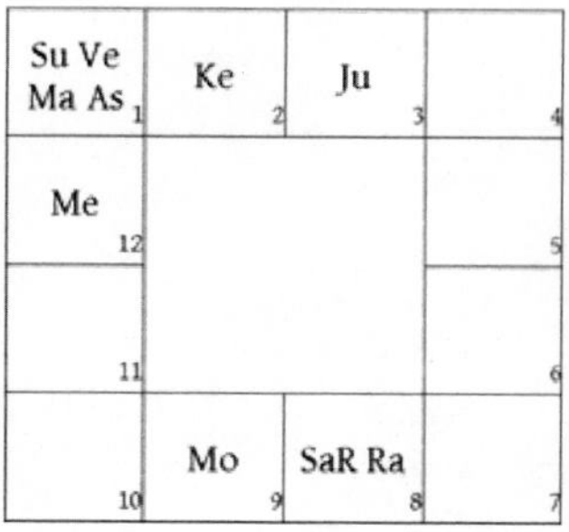

April 2013

S	M	T	W	T	F	S
	1	2	3	4	5	6
7	8	9	10	11	12	13
14	15	16	17	18	19	20
21	22	23	24	25	26	27
28	29	30				

Sunday
7

Śatabhiṣā			7:02
K 13			26:20
Śukla			17:20
Gara			14:34
Vanija			26:20
Rāhu Kālam	17:59	-	19:35

Monday
8

Pūrva Bhādrapadā			7:13
K 14			26:13
Brahma			16:00
Viṣṭi			14:13
Śakuni			26:13
Rāhu Kālam	8:20	-	9:56
Moon: Pisces			1:08

Tuesday
9 ●

Uttara Bhādrapadā			7:51
Āmāvasyā			26:35
Mahendra			15:01
Catuṣpada			14:20
Nāga			26:35
Rāhu Kālam	16:21	-	18:00
Mercury: Pisces			13:26

Wednesday
10

Revatī			8:58
Ś 1			27:28
Vaidhṛti			14:27
Kiṃsthughna			14:58
Bava			27:28
Rāhu Kālam	13:09	-	14:46
Moon: Aries			8:58
Venus: Aries			5:00

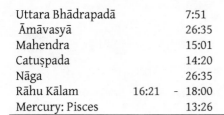

Thursday
11

Aśviṇī			10:36
Ś 2			28:53
Viṣkambha			14:18
Bālava			16:07
Kaulava			28:53
Rāhu Kālam	14:46	-	16:24

Friday
12

Bharaṇī			12:44
Ś 3			Full Night
Prīti			14:32
Taitila			17:47
Gara			Full Night
Rāhu Kālam	11:31	-	13:08
Moon: Taurus			19:20
Mars: Aries			7:07

Saturday
13

Kṛttikā			15:18
Ś 3			6:47
Āyuṣmān			15:07
Gara			6:47
Vanija			19:53
Rāhu Kālam	9:52	-	11:30
Sun: Aries			12:53

Tamiḷ New Year
Puṇya Kāla: 9:25 - 16:23 •

April 2013

S	M	T	W	T	F	S
	1	2	3	4	5	6
7	8	9	10	11	12	13
14	15	16	17	18	19	20
21	22	23	24	25	26	27
28	29	30				

As Su Ma Ve 1	Ke 2	Ju 3	4
Mo Me 12			5
11			6
10	9	SaR Ra 8	7

May 2013

S	M	T	W	T	F	S
			1	2	3	4
5	6	7	8	9	10	11
12	13	14	15	16	17	18
19	20	21	22	23	24	25
26	27	28	29	30	31	

First day of Aries → (first sign in zodiac)

Sunday

14

new years

Vishu

Rohinī			18:12	
Ś 4			9:04	
Saubhāgya			15:58	
Viṣṭi			9:04	
Bava			22:19	
Rāhu Kālam	18:03	-	19:41	Viṣu

Monday

15

Mṛgaśīrṣa			21:15	
Ś 5			11:35	
Śobhana			16:56	
Bālava			11:35	
Kaulava			24:52	
Rāhu Kālam	8:12	-	9:50	
Moon: Gemini			7:43	Income Taxes Due

Tuesday

16

Ārdrā			24:16
Ś 6			14:08
Atigaṇḍa			17:55
Taitila			14:08
Gara			27:20
Rāhu Kālam	16:25	-	18:04

Wednesday

17

Punarvasu			27:00
Ś 7			16:29
Sukarmā			18:43
Vanija			16:29
Viṣṭi			29:30
Rāhu Kālam	13:07	-	14:46
Moon: Cancer			20:21

Thursday

18

Puṣyā			29:16	
Ś 8			18:24	
Dhṛti			19:12	
Bava			18:24	
Bālava			Full Night	
Rāhu Kālam	14:46	-	16:26	

Friday

19

Āśleṣā			Full Night	
Ś 9			19:44	
Śūla			19:13	
Bālava			7:09	
Kaulava			19:44	
Rāhu Kālam	11:27	-	13:07	Hindu New Year • Śrī Rāma Jayantī

Saturday

20

Āśleṣā			6:55	
Ś 10			20:22	
Gaṇḍa			18:41	
Taitila			8:09	
Gara			20:22	
Rāhu Kālam	9:46	-	11:26	
Moon: Leo			6:55	Norvin E. Smith Jr. Day (Hawai'i)

April 2013

S	M	T	W	T	F	S
	1	2	3	4	5	6
7	8	9	10	11	12	13
14	15	16	17	18	19	20
21	22	23	24	25	26	27
28	29	30				

Me 12	Su Ma Ve As Ke 1	Mo Ju 2	3
11			4
10			5
9	8	SaR Ra 7	6

May 2013

S	M	T	W	T	F	S
			1	2	3	4
5	6	7	8	9	10	11
12	13	14	15	16	17	18
19	20	21	22	23	24	25
26	27	28	29	30	31	

Sunday
21

Maghā			7:49	
Ś 11			20:13	
Vṛddhi			17:34	
Vanija			8:23	
Viṣṭi			20:13	
Rāhu Kālam	18:07	-	19:48	

Monday
22

Pūrva Phalguṇī			7:59	
Ś 12			19:19	
Dhruva			15:50	
Bava			7:51	
Bālava			19:19	
Rāhu Kālam	8:04	-	9:45	
Moon: Virgo			13:55	Earth Day

Tuesday
23

Uttara Phalguṇī			7:27	
Hasta			30:16	
Ś 13			17:44	
Vyāghāta			13:33	
Kaulava			6:36	
Taitila			17:44	
Gara			28:43	
Rāhu Kālam	16:28	-	18:09	Mahāvīr Jayantī

Wednesday
24

Citrā			28:35	
Ś 14			15:34	
Harṣaṇa			10:47	
Vanija			15:34	
Viṣṭi			26:18	
Rāhu Kālam	13:06	-	14:47	
Moon: Libra			17:29	

Thursday ○

25

Svāti			26:32	
Pūrṇimā			12:57	
Vajra			7:37	
Siddhi			28:10	
Bava			12:57	
Bālava			23:30	
Rāhu Kālam	14:47	-	16:29	Hanumān Jayantī

Friday

26

Viśākhā			24:16
K 1			10:00
Vyatīpāta			24:32
Kaulava			10:00
Taitila			20:28
Rāhu Kālam	11:24	-	13:05
Moon: Scorpio			18:51

Saturday

27

Anurādha			21:54
K 2			6:54
K 3			27:45
Vāriyān			20:51
Gara			6:54
Vanija			17:19
Viṣṭi			27:45
Rāhu Kālam	9:41	-	11:23

April 2013

S	M	T	W	T	F	S
	1	2	3	4	5	6
7	8	9	10	11	12	13
14	15	16	17	18	19	20
21	22	23	24	25	26	27
28	29	30				

Me 12	Ma Su Ve Ke As 1	Ju 2	3
11			4
10			Mo 5
9	8	SaR Ra 7	6

May 2013

S	M	T	W	T	F	S
			1	2	3	4
5	6	7	8	9	10	11
12	13	14	15	16	17	18
19	20	21	22	23	24	25
26	27	28	29	30	31	

Sunday

28

Jyeṣṭhā			19:36
K 4			24:41
Parigha			17:12
Bava			14:12
Bālava			24:41
Rāhu Kālam	18:12	-	19:54
Moon: Sagittarius			19:36
Mercury: Aries			5:59

Monday

29

Mūla			17:29
K 5			21:50
Śiva			13:41
Kaulava			11:14
Taitila			21:50
Rāhu Kālam	7:57	-	9:40

Tuesday

30

Pūrvāṣāḍhā			15:39
K 6			19:17
Siddha			10:24
Gara			8:31
Vanija			19:17
Viṣṭi			30:10
Rāhu Kālam	16:30	-	18:13
Moon: Capricorn			21:15

Wednesday

1

Uttarāṣāḍhā			14:12	
K 7			17:08	
Sādhya			7:24	
Śubha			28:46	
Bava			17:08	
Bālava			28:14	
Rāhu Kālam	13:05	-	14:48	Beltaine

Thursday

2

Śravaṇa		13:12
K 8		15:26
Śukla		26:31
Kaulava		15:26
Taitila		26:46
Rāhu Kālam	14:48 -	16:31

Friday

3

Dhaniṣṭhā		12:41
K 9		14:14
Brahma		24:41
Gara		14:14
Vanija		25:49
Rāhu Kālam	11:21 -	13:05
Moon: Aquarius		0:52

Saturday

4

Śatabhiṣā		12:40
K 10		13:33
Mahendra		23:15
Viṣṭi		13:33
Bava		25:24
Rāhu Kālam	9:37 -	11:21
Venus: Libra		11:57

April 2013

S	M	T	W	T	F	S
	1	2	3	4	5	6
7	8	9	10	11	12	13
14	15	16	17	18	19	20
21	22	23	24	25	26	27
28	29	30				

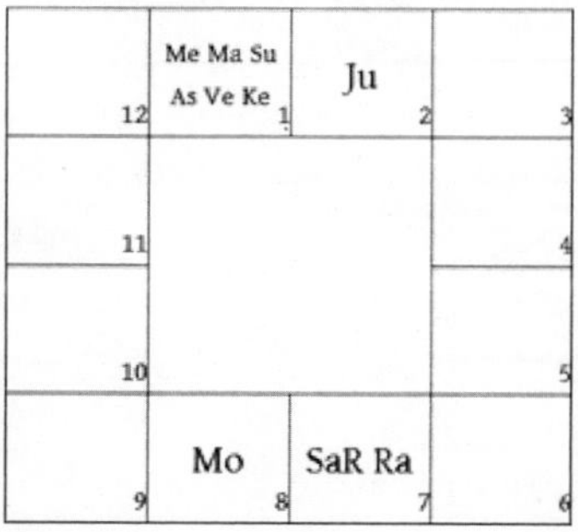

May 2013

S	M	T	W	T	F	S
			1	2	3	4
5	6	7	8	9	10	11
12	13	14	15	16	17	18
19	20	21	22	23	24	25
26	27	28	29	30	31	

Sunday

5

Pūrva Bhādrapadā		13:10	
K 11		13:22	
Vaidhṛti		22:14	
Bālava		13:22	
Kaulava		25:29	
Rāhu Kālam	18:17	- 20:01	
Moon: Pisces		7:00	Cinco de Mayo

Monday

6

Uttara Bhādrapadā		14:10
K 12		13:42
Viṣkambha		21:36
Taitila		13:42
Gara		26:03
Rāhu Kālam	7:51	- 9:36

Tuesday

7

Revatī		15:37
K 13		14:31
Prīti		21:21
Vanija		14:31
Viṣṭi		27:06
Rāhu Kālam	16:33	- 18:18
Moon: Aries		15:37

Wednesday

8

Aśvinī		17:31
K 14		15:47
Āyuṣmān		21:26
Śakuni		15:47
Catuṣpada		28:35
Rāhu Kālam	13:04	- 14:49

Thursday ●

9

Bharaṇī			19:49
Āmāvasyā			17:28
Saubhāgya			21:50
Nāga			17:28
Kiṃsthughna			Full Night
Rāhu Kālam	14:49	-	16:34

Friday

10

Kṛttikā			22:27
Ś 1			19:30
Śobhana			22:29
Kiṃsthughna			6:26
Bava			19:30
Rāhu Kālam	11:19	-	13:04
Moon: Taurus			2:27

Saturday

11

Rohinī			25:20
Ś 2			21:48
Atigaṇḍa			23:21
Bālava			8:37
Kaulava			21:48
Rāhu Kālam	9:33	-	11:19

May 2013

S	M	T	W	T	F	S
			1	2	3	4
5	6	7	8	9	10	11
12	13	14	15	16	17	18
19	20	21	22	23	24	25
26	27	28	29	30	31	

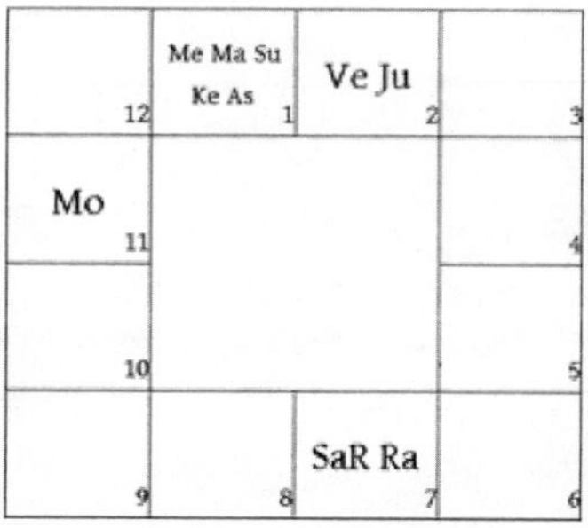

June 2013

S	M	T	W	T	F	S
						1
2	3	4	5	6	7	8
9	10	11	12	13	14	15
16	17	18	19	20	21	22
23	24	25	26	27	28	29
30						

Sunday
12

Mṛgaśīrṣa		28:23	
Ś 3		24:17	
Sukarmā		24:20	
Taitila		11:02	
Gara		24:17	
Rāhu Kālam	18:21	- 20:07	
Moon: Gemini		14:51	
Mercury: Taurus		20:08	Akṣāya Tritīyā • Mother's Day

Monday
13

Ārdrā		Full Night	
Ś 4		26:49	
Dhṛti		25:22	
Vanija		13:33	
Viṣṭi		26:49	
Rāhu Kālam	7:46	- 9:32	Ramanuja Jayantī

Tuesday
14

Ārdrā		7:26	
Ś 5		29:13	
Śūla		26:18	
Bava		16:03	
Bālava		29:13	
Rāhu Kālam	16:36	- 18:22	Śaṅkāra Jayantī
Sun: Taurus		9:46	Puṇya Kāla: 2:13 - 9:46

Wednesday
15

Punarvasu		10:21	
Ś 6		Full Night	
Gaṇḍa		27:03	
Kaulava		18:20	
Taitila		Full Night	
Rāhu Kālam	13:04	- 14:50	
Moon: Cancer		3:39	

Thursday

16

Puṣyā			12:57
Ś 6			7:20
Vṛddhi			27:27
Taitila			7:20
Gara			20:13
Rāhu Kālam	14:51	-	16:37

Friday

17

Āṣleśā			15:04
Ś 7			8:58
Dhruva			27:23
Vanija			8:58
Viṣṭi			21:34
Rāhu Kālam	11:17	-	13:04
Moon: Leo			15:04

Saturday

18

Maghā			16:33	
Ś 8			9:59	
Vyāghāta			26:47	
Bava			9:59	
Bālava			22:14	
Rāhu Kālam	9:30	-	11:17	Armed Forces Day

May 2013

S	M	T	W	T	F	S
			1	2	3	4
5	6	7	8	9	10	11
12	13	14	15	16	17	18
19	20	21	22	23	24	25
26	27	28	29	30	31	

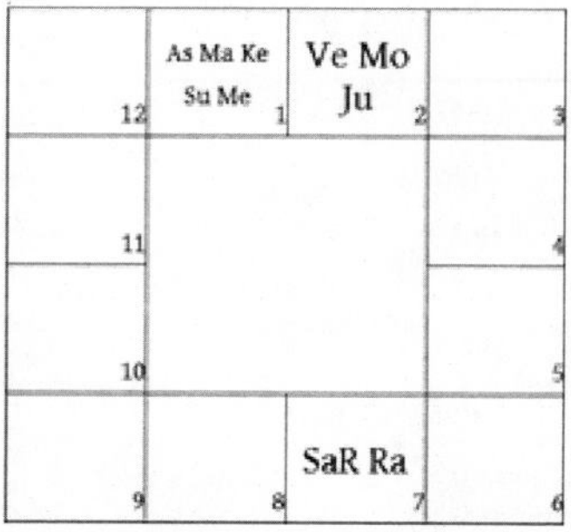

June 2013

S	M	T	W	T	F	S
						1
2	3	4	5	6	7	8
9	10	11	12	13	14	15
16	17	18	19	20	21	22
23	24	25	26	27	28	29
30						

Sunday 19

Pūrva Phalguṇī			17:19	
Ś 9			10:17	
Harṣaṇa			25:35	
Kaulava			10:17	
Taitila			22:08	
Rāhu Kālam	18:26	-	20:13	
Moon: Virgo			23:23	Pentecost

Monday 20

Uttara Phalguṇī			17:18	
Ś 10			9:48	
Vajra			23:45	
Gara			9:48	
Vanija			21:16	
Rāhu Kālam	7:42	-	9:29	Pentecost Monday

Tuesday 21

Hasta			16:33
Ś 11			8:32
Siddhi			21:19
Viṣṭi			8:32
Bava			19:38
Rāhu Kālam	16:39	-	18:27

Wednesday 22

Citrā			15:06
Ś 12			6:33
Ś 13			27:57
Vyatīpāta			18:21
Bālava			6:33
Kaulava			17:20
Taitila			27:57
Rāhu Kālam	13:04	-	14:52
Moon: Libra			3:54
Mars: Taurus			20:43

Thursday
23

Svāti			13:04
Ś 14			24:51
Varīyān			14:55
Gara			14:28
Vanija			24:51
Rāhu Kālam	14:52	-	16:40

Friday
24

Viśākhā			10:37
Pūrṇimā			21:24
Parigha			11:07
Viṣṭi			11:10
Bava			21:24
Rāhu Kālam	11:16	-	13:04
Moon: Scorpio			5:15

Saturday
25

Anurādha			7:52
Jyeṣṭhā			29:01
K 1			17:46
Śiva			7:06
Siddha			26:59
Bālava			7:36
Kaulava			17:46
Taitila			27:55
Rāhu Kālam	9:28	-	11:16

May 2013

S	M	T	W	T	F	S
			1	2	3	4
5	6	7	8	9	10	11
12	13	14	15	16	17	18
19	20	21	22	23	24	25
26	27	28	29	30	31	

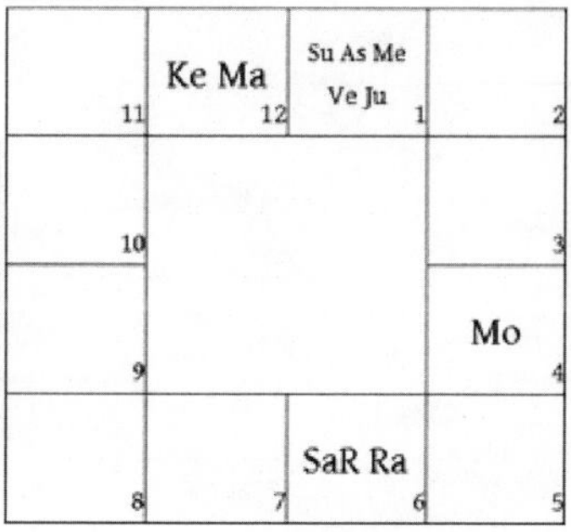

June 2013

S	M	T	W	T	F	S
						1
2	3	4	5	6	7	8
9	10	11	12	13	14	15
16	17	18	19	20	21	22
23	24	25	26	27	28	29
30						

Sunday

26

Mūla		26:12	
K 2		14:05	
Sādhya		22:55	
Gara		14:05	
Vanija		24:17	
Rāhu Kālam	18:30	- 20:18	
Moon: Sagittarius		5:01	

Monday

27

Pūrvāṣāḍhā		23:39	
K 3		10:32	
Śubha		19:00	
Viṣṭi		10:32	
Bava		20:52	
Rāhu Kālam	7:39	- 9:28	
Mercury: Gemini		12:10	Memorial Day

Tuesday

28

Uttarāṣāḍhā		21:28	
K 4		7:17	
K 5		28:27	
Śukla		15:23	
Bālava		7:17	
Kaulava		17:48	
Taitila		28:27	
Rāhu Kālam	16:42	- 18:31	
Venus: Gemini		12:10	

Wednesday

29

Śravaṇa		19:47	
K 6		26:10	
Brahma		12:09	
Gara		15:14	
Vanija		26:10	
Rāhu Kālam	13:05	- 14:54	

Thursday
30

Dhaniṣṭhā		18:44
K 7		24:31
Mahendra		9:25
Viṣṭi		13:16
Bava		24:31
Rāhu Kālam	14:54 -	16:43
Jupiter: Gemini		18:18

Friday
31

Śatabhiṣā		18:21
K 8		23:35
Vaidhṛti		7:13
Viṣkambha		29:35
Bālava		11:58
Kaulava		23:35
Rāhu Kālam	11:16 -	13:05

Saturday
1

Pūrva Bhādrapadā		18:41
K 9		23:20
Prīti		28:31
Taitila		11:22
Gara		23:20
Rāhu Kālam	9:27 -	11:16
Moon: Pisces		12:32

May 2013

S	M	T	W	T	F	S
			1	2	3	4
5	6	7	8	9	10	11
12	13	14	15	16	17	18
19	20	21	22	23	24	25
26	27	28	29	30	31	

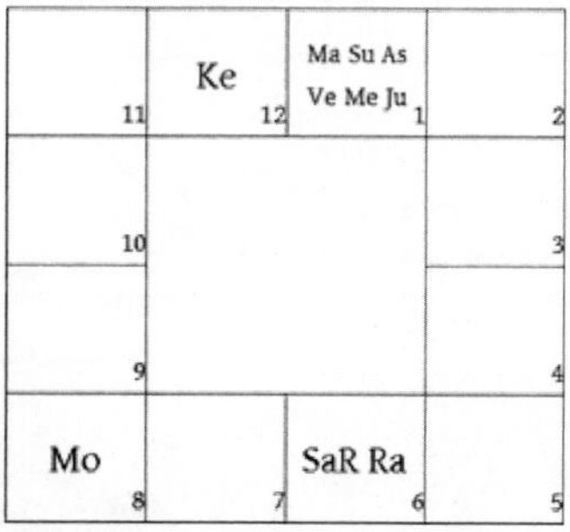

June 2013

S	M	T	W	T	F	S
						1
2	3	4	5	6	7	8
9	10	11	12	13	14	15
16	17	18	19	20	21	22
23	24	25	26	27	28	29
30						

Sunday
2

Uttara Bhādrapadā			19:41
K 10			23:46
Āyuṣman			27:58
Vanija			11:28
Viṣṭi			23:46
Rāhu Kālam	18:34	-	20:23

Monday
3

Revatī			21:17
K 11			24:48
Saubhāgya			27:53
Bava			12:13
Bālava			24:48
Rāhu Kālam	7:37	-	9:27
Mercury: Aries			21:17

Tuesday
4

Aśvinī			23:23
K 12			26:21
Śobhana			28:11
Kaulava			13:31
Taitila			26:21
Rāhu Kālam	16:45	-	18:35

Wednesday
5

Bharaṇī			25:53
K 13			28:17
Atigaṇḍa			28:47
Gara			15:17
Vanija			28:17
Rāhu Kālam	13:06	-	14:56

Thursday

6

Kṛttikā			28:40
K 14			Full Night
Sukarmā			29:35
Viṣṭi			17:23
Śakuni			Full Night
Rāhu Kālam	14:56	-	16:46
Moon: Taurus			8:34

Friday

7

Rohinī			Full Night
K 14			6:31
Dhṛti			Full Night
Śakuni			6:31
Catuṣpada			19:43
Rāhu Kālam	11:17	-	13:07

Saturday

8

Rohinī			7:39
Āmāvasyā			8:56
Dhṛti			6:33
Nāgava			8:56
Kiṃsthughna			22:10
Rāhu Kālam	9:27	-	11:17
Moon: Gemini			21:10

May 2013

S	M	T	W	T	F	S
			1	2	3	4
5	6	7	8	9	10	11
12	13	14	15	16	17	18
19	20	21	22	23	24	25
26	27	28	29	30	31	

Mo 11	Ke 12	Ma Su As 1	Ju Ve Me 2
10			3
9			4
8	7	SaR Ra 6	5

June 2013

S	M	T	W	T	F	S
						1
2	3	4	5	6	7	8
9	10	11	12	13	14	15
16	17	18	19	20	21	22
23	24	25	26	27	28	29
30						

Sunday

9

Mṛgaśīrṣa			10:42
Ś 1			11:25
Śūla			7:35
Bava			11:25
Bālava			24:40
Rāhu Kālam	18:37	-	20:27

Monday

10

Ārdrā			13:45
Ś 2			13:54
Gaṇḍa			8:36
Kaulava			13:54
Taitila			27:06
Rāhu Kālam	7:37	-	9:27

Tuesday

11

Punarvasu			16:41
Ś 3			16:16
Vṛddhi			9:34
Gara			16:16
Vanija			29:23
Rāhu Kālam	16:48	-	18:38
Moon: Cancer			9:58

Wednesday

12

Puṣyā			19:24
Ś 4			18:25
Dhruva			10:23
Viṣṭi			18:25
Bava			Full Night
Rāhu Kālam	13:07	-	14:58

Thursday

13

Āśleṣā		21:47
Ś 5		20:12
Vyāghāta		10:57
Bava		7:22
Bālava		20:12
Rāhu Kālam	14:58 -	16:48
Moon: Leo		21:47

Friday

14

Maghā		23:42	
Ś 6		21:32	
Harṣaṇa		11:12	
Kaulava		8:56	
Taitila		21:32	
Rāhu Kālam	11:17 -	13:08	
Sun: Gemini		16:20	Flag Day • Puṇya Kāla: 16:20 - 24:16

Saturday

15

Pūrva Phalguṇī		25:02
Ś 7		22:16
Vajra		11:02
Gara		9:59
Vanija		22:16
Rāhu Kālam	9:27 -	11:18

May 2013

S	M	T	W	T	F	S
			1	2	3	4
5	6	7	8	9	10	11
12	13	14	15	16	17	18
19	20	21	22	23	24	25
26	27	28	29	30	31	

11	Ke 12	Ma As Su 1	Ju Mo Ve Me 2
10			3
9			4
8	7	SaR Ra 6	5

June 2013

S	M	T	W	T	F	S
						1
2	3	4	5	6	7	8
9	10	11	12	13	14	15
16	17	18	19	20	21	22
23	24	25	26	27	28	29
30						

Sunday
16

Uttara Phalguṇī			25:43	
Ś 8			22:20	
Siddhi			10:22	
Viṣṭi			10:23	
Bava			22:20	
Rāhu Kālam	18:40	-	20:30	
Moon: Virgo			7:16	Father's Day

Monday
17

Hasta			25:39
Ś 9			21:39
Vyatīpāta			9:08
Bālava			10:05
Kaulava			21:39
Rāhu Kālam	7:37	-	9:27

Tuesday
18

Citrā			24:51
Ś 10			20:14
Varīyān			7:18
Parigha			28:52
Taitila			9:02
Gara			20:14
Rāhu Kālam	16:50	-	18:40
Moon: Libra			13:21

Wednesday
19

Svāti			23:22
Ś 11			18:05
Śiva			25:53
Vanija			7:15
Viṣṭi			18:05
Bava			28:47
Rāhu Kālam	13:09	-	14:59

Thursday
20

Viśākhā			21:16
Ś 12			15:20
Siddha			22:24
Bālava			15:20
Kaulava			25:45
Rāhu Kālam	15:00	-	16:50
Moon: Scorpio			15:50

Summer Solstice 22:04

Friday
21

Anurādha			18:41
Ś 13			12:03
Sādhya			18:31
Taitila			12:03
Gara			22:15
Rāhu Kālam	11:19	-	13:09

Saturday ○
22

Jyeṣṭhā			15:46
Ś 14			8:24
Pūrṇimā			28:32
Śubha			14:22
Vanija			8:24
Viṣṭi			18:29
Bava			28:32
Rāhu Kālam	9:27	-	11:18
Moon: Sagittarius			15:46
Venus: Cancer			12:29

May 2013

S	M	T	W	T	F	S
			1	2	3	4
5	6	7	8	9	10	11
12	13	14	15	16	17	18
19	20	21	22	23	24	25
26	27	28	29	30	31	

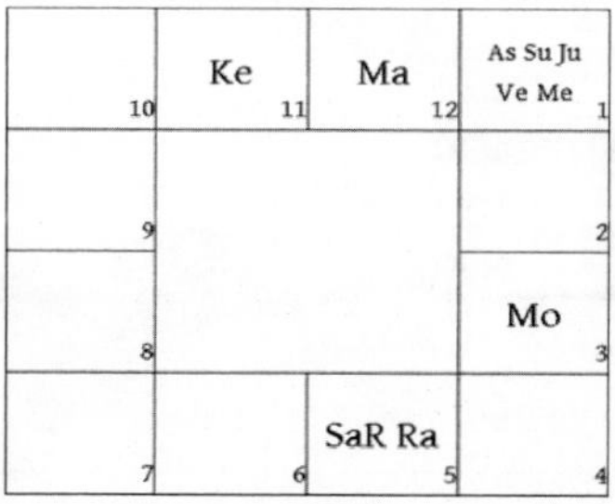

June 2013

S	M	T	W	T	F	S
						1
2	3	4	5	6	7	8
9	10	11	12	13	14	15
16	17	18	19	20	21	22
23	24	25	26	27	28	29
30						

Sunday
23

Mūla			12:43
K 1			24:38
Śukla			10:05
Bālava			14:34
Kaulava			24:38
Rāhu Kālam	18:41	-	20:32

Monday
24

Pūrvāṣāḍhā			9:42
K 2			20:53
Brahma			5:49
Mahendra			25:42
Taitila			10:43
Gara			20:53
Rāhu Kālam	7:38	-	9:29
Moon: Capricorn			14:58

Tuesday
25

Uttarāṣāḍhā			6:54
Śravaṇa			28:32
K 3			17:27
Vaidhṛti			21:54
Vanija			7:07
Viṣṭi			17:27
Bava			27:54
Rāhu Kālam	16:51	-	18:42

Wednesday
26

Dhaniṣṭhā			26:44
K 4			14:30
Viṣkambha			18:32
Bālava			14:30
Kaulava			25:16
Rāhu Kālam	13:10	-	15:01
Moon: Aquarius			15:33

Thursday

27

Śatabhiṣā			25:40
K 5			12:12
Prīti			15:44
Taitila			12:12
Gara			23:20
Rāhu Kālam	15:01	-	16:51

Friday

28

Pūrva Bhādrapadā			25:21
K 6			10:40
Āyuṣman			13:33
Vanija			10:40
Viṣṭi			22:12
Rāhu Kālam	11:20	-	13:11
Moon: Pisces			19:20

Saturday

29

Uttara Bhādrapadā			25:52
K 7			9:56
Saubhāgya			12:02
Bava			9:56
Bālava			21:53
Rāhu Kālam	9:30	-	11:21

May 2013

S	M	T	W	T	F	S
			1	2	3	4
5	6	7	8	9	10	11
12	13	14	15	16	17	18
19	20	21	22	23	24	25
26	27	28	29	30	31	

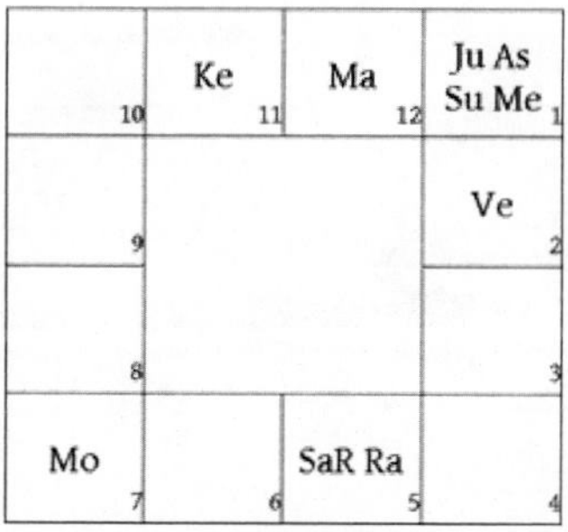

June 2013

S	M	T	W	T	F	S
						1
2	3	4	5	6	7	8
9	10	11	12	13	14	15
16	17	18	19	20	21	22
23	24	25	26	27	28	29
30						

Chapter Four

~

SUMMER

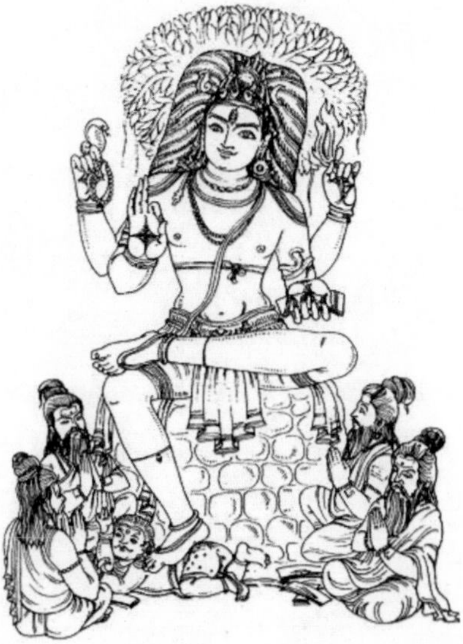

Dakṣiṇāmūrti and the Four Sons of Brahmā

~

Part 1

Many, many years ago, Lord Brahmā, the God of creation, started to become restless and tired. He had been creating world after world and creature after creature – from the smallest ant to the largest elephant, for a long period of time. A seemingly endless stream of delightful and wonderful creations had been manifest by him and each was unique and imbued with the spark of divinity. In the midst of all of this wonderful creating, a desire began to grow in the innermost layer of Lord Brahmā's heart. This feeling grew from a curious tingling to a noticeable twitch and eventually culminated into a deep pang. Finally, one evening after his duties had been finished, Lord Brahmā ascended his bejeweled throne and let out a large sigh of longing from each of his four heads.

Saraswatī, Lord Brahmā's ever devoted wife and faithful companion, noticed this and approached him.

"Alas my Lord, what has been troubling you as of late? I know that there is something in your heart that you desire and if it is within my power, I want no more than to obtain it for you. Please, tell me so that I can serve you my Lord!"

"It is nothing my dear, nothing with which to trouble you." Lord Brahmā replied.

But Saraswatī Mā knew in her heart that something was off and she felt deeply pained to see her resplendent husband fretting.

"You have been working *so* hard lately. Why don't you take a break from your job of creating, my darling? Before you started the act of creation the world was perfect, while you've been creating the world has remained perfect and if you were to take a short break, the world will remain perfect. Besides my Lord," Saraswatī continued, "You mustn't allow Lord Viṣṇu and Lord Śiva to fall behind on their duties of sustaining and dissolution."

Lord Brahmā sat for a moment, pondering his loving wife's proposal. "Well, I am finding this business of dreaming up and breathing life into an ever expanding array of creations growing a bit repetitive. My dear, you indeed are correct. What I need is a vacation."

Saraswatī's silk sari seemed to glow like the full moon as she approached the golden throne on which Lord Brahmā sat. "Yes, what you need my dear, is a chance to retreat from this magnificent creation of yours and go inward for some time. Remember many years ago when we spent those countless days in meditation on the Self and the untold satisfaction that accompanied them?" Saraswatī Mā paused as she tenderly took hold of Lord Brahmā's hand. "Yes my Lord, this is exactly what you need. Let us return to planet Earth, to the snow crested Himālayās, to spend some time immersing our minds once again, into the Source of All."

"Parāśaktī, as usual, you could not be more correct. Let us set off for the Himalāyās at once. But..." Lord Brahmā paused, "Let me first do one thing. I shall create a few divine beings with pure intention who will continue this needed work of creation while we are on our sojourn."

"Very well, my Lord. I will retire to our chambers to arrange provisions for the trip."

And so it was decided. Lord Brahmā and his celestial wife would retire to the heavenly Himālayās to practice meditation in the still solitude of the mountains and valleys there. As planned, Lord Brahmā set about creating four noble-minded souls that he could entrust with the task of manifesting new creations while he took his retreat.

"Let me think for a moment," Lord Brahmā thought to himself. "These four beings that I will give my powers to, they mustn't be ordinary beings. They must not be too young, they must be endowed with eternal life, they must be ever joyful and they must be of divine birth. I've got it! They will be divine sages and I will name them Sanaka, Sanat Kumāra, Sānanda and Sanatsujāta; they will be masters of all 64 branches of divine knowledge and have the sole intention of living to benefit the worlds."

Within the amount of time that occurs between two successive thoughts, it was so. Standing before Lord Brahmā were four radiant sages.

"Namaste, father." They spoke with bowed heads.

"Namaste, my sons," Lord Brahmā said as he smiled and pulled them into his mighty arms. "You, my dear ones, will be assigned with a marvelous and wonderful task. You will continue the role of Creator while I retire to the Himālayās to practice austerities and meditation."

A benign smile crossed their faces. Sanatsujāta spoke, "Father, our sincere salutations for bringing us into the world but I think that you are mistaken. You see, having mastered the 64 divine arts, we intimately know every aspect of your creation. Now, you must understand, we desire not to create more karma for ourselves by taking on your duties as Creator and being responsible for the resulting creations. Rather, we desire to know the very essence of life and to pursue *ātma jñāna*, knowledge of the Self."

Taken by surprise, Lord Brahmā managed to stammer out, "This cannot be! I have created you four, in all of your divine glory, to assume my duties as Creator, while I take to the mountains with Saraswatī Devī to practice meditation."

"Actually, Worshipful One, we feel that your plan will have to be indefinitely postponed. We four now ask your blessing to take leave of you, so that we may seek a spiritual teacher who will initiate us into that excellent Path of Ultimate Liberation, the path of Knowledge of the Self."

Before Lord Brahmā had a chance to realize the implications of their words, he had raised his hand in blessing and the four sagely brothers bowed low and turned to leave.

"Wait ... sons!" Brahmā exclaimed.

Sanaka spoke as he was crossing the threshold of the room. "My Lord, you are our father as well as the innermost Self of all. Please know that we simply must fulfill our duty so that will also benefit all of creation. We have but one desire left and that is for Self-realization.

Some time later, Saraswatī entered the room to see her husband sitting despondently on his throne.

"Lord, I have packed your meditation mat, prayer rosary and some basic supplies for our journey. What is the matter that you look so somber? Is there something more that you need?"

"No, my devoted wife. You have once again exceeded my expectations. It's only that ... well, you see ... the four pious sons that I created to relieve me temporarily of my duties ... have left!"

Shocked, Saraswatī exclaimed, "My Lord, how can this be? What about our plans and your needed solitude?"

"It is true Devī. What to do now?"

Instantly regaining her serene composure, Saraswatī approached her perplexed husband and took his hands in hers. Speaking softly to his heart, she said, "Oh Brahmā, please do not worry. I should have had the foresight to know that if you were to create perfect offspring who were endowed with knowledge of the 64 divine arts, they would not tolerate creating any new karmas. Because of the perfect knowledge regarding the arts, they have taken to pursuit of *that* knowledge which bestows understanding of the very Self of all." She paused, and then continued. "Rather than being forlorned about this unexpected turn of events, I would like to suggest to you that you simply continue to practice your duties as Creator. This job is what karma has assigned to you and we mustn't long for that duty which isn't naturally ours. To relax and meditate in the majestic Himālayās for countless years just wouldn't be proper. It is better, my Lord, for you to do your duty, even if you are tired, than pursue the duty of another just because it feels good. Your sons are the ones who should be following a meditative and contemplative way of life. Why don't we stay here? Allow me to continue to serve you and this way you can continue the act of creating. This will enable your sons their leave to find their noble lot in life."

"My dear, dear Goddess, again, how can I argue with you? You are as compassionate as you are beautiful. Then it is decided, we will stay here, continuing our duties and allow nature to take its course."

And so it was. Brahmā stayed in his abode, continuing to create, while his four noble sons started their journey on the path of Self Knowledge.

To be continued...

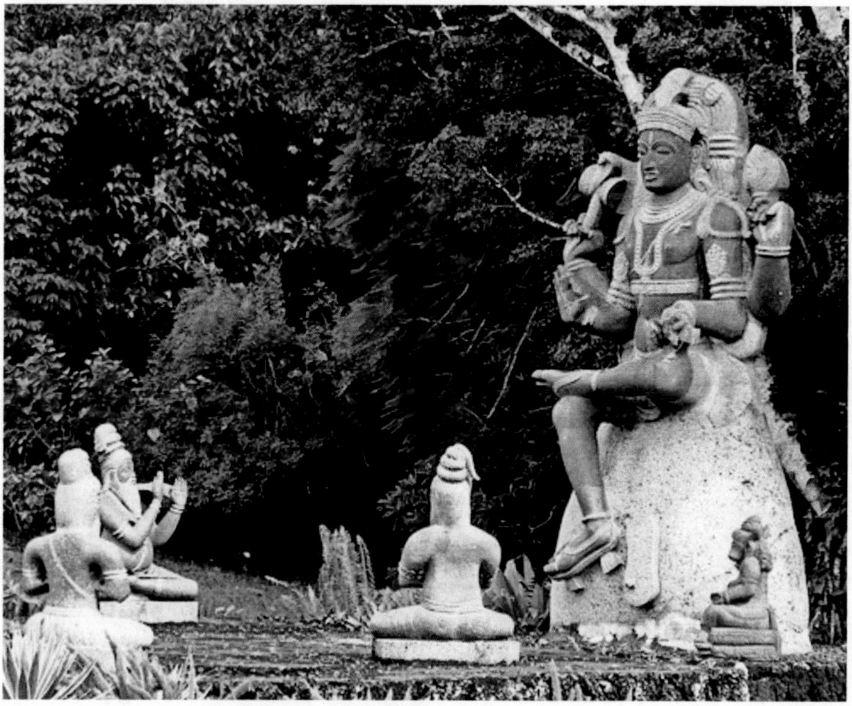

Dakṣiṇāmūrti image courtesy the Kauai Hindu Monastery

Hasta Sāmudrika Śāstra

~

The Fire Hand

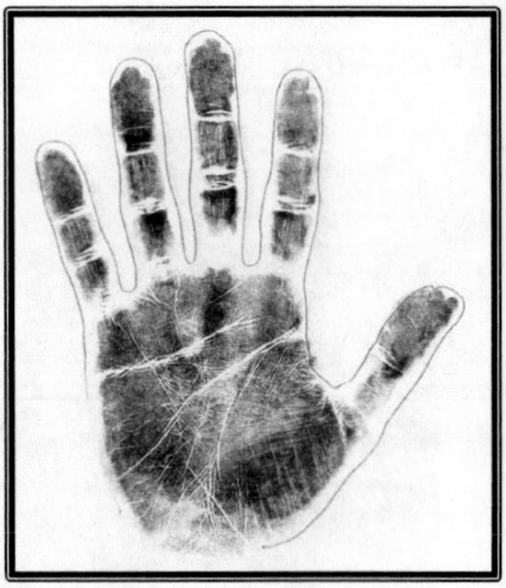

Summer brings warmth, activity, extroversion and expansion. Just as the Sun burns, pulsing with energy, so the hands dominated by the fire element reflect a personality that is ardent, expressive, radiant and brimming with enthusiasm. Fire-handed people are adventurous, friendly and exciting to be with. They thrive on getting things done and are often passionate about bringing change to the world.

Palm

The typical fire hand has a rectangular palm. That means that when you look at the palm, it appears more like a rectangle than a square. Rectangles are a shape that induces movement and the fire-handed person is dynamic. Fire types are energetic and love physical activity, especially when that activity is challenging or competitive; they tend to be always on the go. This fiery vibrancy can sometimes make it difficult for fire-hand types to stick to routines and habits. They would rather go have a new adventure!

Fingers

The fingers of the typical fire hand are short in relation to the palm. To determine finger length, measure and compare the length of the middle finger to the length of the palm. If the finger length is less than ¾ than that of the palm then consider the fingers as short.

Finger length is indicative of how much time a person spontaneously spends thinking about things and how attentive to detail they are. This is one of the few counter-intuitive categories in hand analysis. Most people think that the shorter the fingers and the smaller the hand, the greater the attention to detail. In fact, the opposite is true: short-fingered people are more likely to grasp a situation quickly and intuitively and gloss over details on their way towards a rapid assessment.

The mind of the short-fingered fire-handed type views things in wide-sweeping fashion. Their natural distaste for detail often gives rise to one of the chief faults of those with fire hands: impatience. Impatience can easily turn into intolerance of those who do not share the fire-type quickness of thought or action. Fire-handed people can literally 'sear' others with their intensity and their sometimes straight-out anger. Conversely, when in balance, that same impetuous nature can ignite enthusiasm and warmth in the hearts of others, bringing the best out of all the fire-handed person interact with.

Just like a burning fire has multiple tongues of flame that flicker with inconsistent energy, a fire-handed person can flicker with enthusiasm at new and exciting things, but then have difficulty sustaining this enthusiasm once the initial fun and joy has subsided. Those with fire hands can readily exemplify the 'jack of all trades and master of none' expression. The inability to commit, focus, and take on the hard work required to master something leads the fire-hand type to move on, sometimes before what they are doing is completed.

The typical fire type dislikes problems that can't be unraveled quickly, as they tend to solve problems intuitively rather than intellectually. How can those of us with fire hands master our element and learn to work with it productively? When we deeply connect to the fire element, we find that fire is innately ambitious. This strong desire to excel, to shine brightly and to be seen by others can be tapped into to curb the more restless aspects of fire and to invite the perseverance and patience necessary to cultivate one's dreams fully and deeply in life. When this process is done successfully, the fire-hand type is capable of the single-minded intensity and focus that leads to great insights and achievements.

Skin Texture

The texture of the skin of the typical fire hand is slightly rough to the touch - but not too much. It is definitely not as rough as the tough skin of the earth hand and far from the silken smoothness of the water hand.

Lines

The palms of a fire hand are traversed by strong, clear lines that are usually reddish in color. Just like the flames of a fire, these lines tend to cross each other at odd angles creating triangles and squares and other geometric shapes. This angularity is reflected in the physiology of the typical fire-handed person (angular features, pointy elbows, etc.) and in the way they move. More than any other type, those with fire hands are prone to accidental mishaps like bumping into things or cutting themselves while chopping vegetables.

Fingerprints

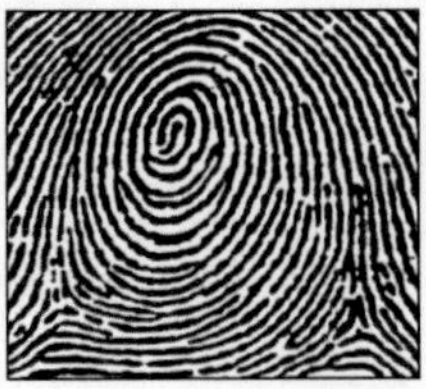

The fingerprint most associated with fire hands is the whorl. Fingerprints can be likened to a sand dune on which varying strengths of wind leave their traces. The whorl is like the most intense trace left by these currents of energy. A whorl, at some point, closes in on itself, forming concentric circles like a bull's eye or a spiral. Note that not all fire hands have whorl fingerprints but if you do find a set of hands with more than four whorls, you are in the clear presence of the fire element.

Whorls, just like their shape suggests, speak to individuality and uniqueness and to a certain intensity. You can count on the fact that a fire-hand type, especially one with a lot of whorls, is very much going to be a person built to march to their own drumbeat, someone who at their core highly values freedom and independence.

Hasta Sāmudrika Śāstra

~

The Heart Line

The heart line is the third-most significant line on the hand, following the life and head lines. It is the uppermost horizontal line on the palm, starting below the little finger and running towards the index finger. It is rare for a palm not to have a heart line, and even then it is generally there in part, merging with the head line into a simian line (see the "Head Line" article for more information about the simian line).

The heart line describes our emotional tendencies, the way we love, and the health of our heart as an organ. It reveals information about all of our relationships, from friendships, to familial relationships, to intimate relationships and marriage. The heart line indicates how open- or closed-hearted we are, to what extent we give to others, and how emotionally demonstrative we are.

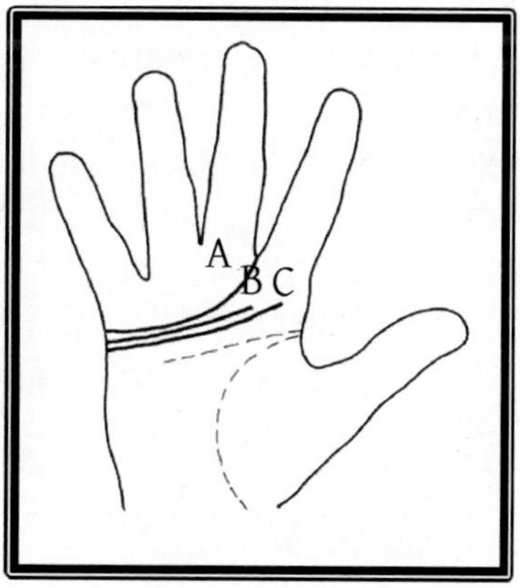

To meaningfully evaluate the heart line, we want to first look at how long it is and then notice how curved, or straight, it is. We can then refine our interpretation by studying the quality of the line. Shown in the diagram above are examples of different heart lines. Line *A* is long and curved upwards, ending between the Jupiter and Saturn fingers. Line *B* is short. Line *C* is average in length, ending below the Jupiter finger.

Length

The average heart line ends somewhere in the area between the index and middle finger. A heart line that reaches to only under the middle finger, also known as the Saturn finger, indicates someone who lacks real emotional involvement and tends to be more rational and controlled emotionally. This short heart line sometimes points to a certain selfishness in the realm of relationship, often manifesting as an incapacity to understand the impact one's actions have on the emotional well-being of others. When it comes to relationships, someone with a short heart line may well wonder foremost: "What's in it for me?"

A long heart line, in contrast, ends somewhere under the index finger (the Jupiter finger) and indicates the ability to love in an idealistic, self-sacrificing way. The longer the heart line, the more mature the person's emotional patterns. The question in the mind of someone with a long heart line is likely to be: "How can I support my partner?"

A very long heart line that reaches the middle of the area under the Jupiter finger or beyond is a clear sign of a humanitarian. This is a person committed to helping others, whose emotions are focused on a larger context, and who gets a lot of their emotional needs met by being of benefit to all.

As we mature emotionally in life, our hearts soften and we become better able to express subtle emotional patterns. This process of heart-energy expansion is sometimes reflected in the hands as small faint thin lines that grow out of the radial (the thumb side) end of the heart line, extending the heart line further in that direction. These subtle lines, or growth tendrils, are a wonderful indicator of the desire to become more giving.

It can be profoundly instructive to examine our own heart lines for an objective view of our emotional character and growth.

Curved or Straight

Whether long or short, the heart line takes one of two main forms: curved or straight.

A person with a straight heart line tends to express their love and affections in a thoughtful manner. Their emotional attitude is less amplified, less demonstrably passionate, and they are more likely to show their feelings through thoughts and words rather than through actions. This makes them appear cool on the emotional front. They usually play a more quiet and receptive role in love affairs, and look for partners who are sincere.

If a straight heart line is also distinctly short (ending before the space under the index and middle finger), the capacity for real loving and caring is diminished, especially if confirmed by other signs like a rigid, hard hand with rough skin.

A person with a curved heart line, on the other hand, will be more demonstrative in their affections—the greater the curvature, the more impulsive the emotional expression. Those with curved heart lines are warm, affectionate, and like to play an active or dominant role in their relationships.

It may seem from the above descriptions that people with straight heart lines are less emotional than people with curved heart lines, but this is not quite the case. They just have different ways of expressing their emotions. The person with a curved heart line is not able to love more or better than one with a straight heart line, or vice versa; they just employ different strategies for managing their emotions and displaying their affections.

While it is easier to find compatibility with those who share our same tendencies around heart matters, and therefore a similar curvature of the heart line, those with mismatched heart lines can get along famously once these emotion-related differences are understood and accepted. A person with a curved heart line, for example, might use a loud voice, gesticulate, and stomp around when in an altercation, while their straight-heart-lined partner sulks, broods, and suffers in silence in a corner. Mismatches only create problems when we do not understand what's really at the core - that we are all different creatures with different strategies around relationships.

Quality

As with all lines, we want the heart line to be clear and well marked. It is normal for the heart line to be somewhat chained and tangled under the little finger, which is actually a good sign for the health of the heart as an organ. But a significantly chained or frayed-looking heart line can indicate one who contends with tangled emotions. Whether the person's convoluted relationship dynamics are dealt with functionally or not depends on how much feathering/chaining there is, and on the overall structure of the hand.

The journey towards healthy and mature emotional expression is a lifelong dance of learning how to pursue our own freedom while simultaneously supporting the freedom of those around us. If in the quest for our own freedom, we make others feel small or insignificant in any way, we reinforce the limited aspect of our being and cut ourselves off from the love of Spirit. If, instead, we move and act in the world in a way that makes others feel respected and free as well, Spirit will rush in to support us just as we support life.

Dakṣiṇāmūrti Stotram
Part III

Verse 6

Rāhugrasta divākar endusadṛśo māyā samācchādanāt
Sanmātraḥ karaṇo pasaṃharaṇato yo'bhūt suṣuptaḥ pumān |
Prāgasvāpsam iti prabodha samaye yaḥ pratya bhijñāyate
Tasmai śrīgurumūrtaye nama idaṃ śrīdakṣiṇāmūrtaye ||

Rāhugrasta – an eclipse; Divākara – that which causes the day, the Sun; Indu – Moon; Sadṛśaḥ - like; Māyā – Illusion; Samācchādanāt – from the complete covering due to māyā; Sanmātraḥ - [sat mātraḥ] –

existence, being alone; Karaṇa – sense organs; Upasaṁharaṇataḥ - withdrawing; Yaḥ - he who; Abhūt – What has not been; Suṣuptaḥ - slept; Pumān – Self

Prāk – before; Asvāpsam – I slept [before]; Iti – verily; Prabodha – of waking up; Samaye – time; Yaḥ - he who; Pratyabhijñāyate – recalls, remembers; Tasmai...

As one whose sense perceptions had completely withdrawn while sleeping and also as when the Sun and Moon are eclipsed, due to the veil of Māyā, the Individual also sees Reality in a dualistic nature, in the form of "this" and "that". At the time of waking up - when the veil of ignorance lifts - these people recall in full awareness "I slept", thus perceiving all as the Self. My deepest salutations to my respected teacher in the form of Dakṣiṇāmūrti.

Verse 7

Bālyādi ṣvapi jāgradādiṣu tathā sarvā svavasthā svapi
Vyāvṛttā svanuvartamāna mahamityantaḥ sphurantaṁ sadā |
Svātmānaṃ prakaṭīkaroti bhajatāṃ yo mudrayā bhadrayā
Tasmai śrīgurūmūrtaye nama idaṃ śrīdakṣaṇoomūrtaye ||

Bālya – childhood; Ādi – etc; Api – and/also; Jāgra – waking, dream, deep sleep state; Tathā – similarly; Sarvāsu – fruitless, barren, vital airs; Avasthāsu – all states of experience; Vyāvṛttāsu – these states of experience negate each other; Anuvartāmāna – that which exists continually Soul; Aham – I; Iti – sayeth; Antar – within; Sphuraṇam – shinning; Sadā – always

Svātmānam – His own Self; Prakaṭī –manifest; karoti – to make manifest, to reveal; Bhajatām – to his devotees and students; Yaḥ - he; Mudrayā Bhadrayā – by the auspicious mudra; Tasmai..

The Self that is always shinning within as "I". It exists continuously in all seasons of life like childhood, adulthood and old age, as well as when one is awake, sleeping, in dreamless sleep and the stage which is beyond - turīya. These experiences by their very nature negate each (when one is young, they are not old, etc.) but the Self is the very thread that connects them all. My deepest salutations to my respected teacher in the form of Dakṣiṇāmūrti, who reveals that Self to his devotees, by means of the auspicious *Cin-Mudra.*

Verse 8

Viśvaṃ paśyati kārya kāraṇatayā svasvāmisambandhataḥ
Śiṣyācārya tayā tathaiva pitṛ putra adyātmanā bhedataḥ |
Svapne jāgrati vā ya eṣa puruṣo māyā paribhrāmitaḥ
Tasmai śrigurumūrtaye nama idaṃ śrīdakṣiṇāmūrtaye ||

Viśvam - the Universe; Paśyati - he sees; Kārya – result; Kāraṇa – cause; Tayā – by, as; Sva – of one's self; Svāmi – master, employer; Sambandhataḥ - relationship; Śiṣya – student; Ācārya – teacher; Tayā – as, in terms of; Tatha eva – similarly, and; Pitra – father; Putra - son; Ādi – etc; Atmanā – again; Bhedataḥ - he who sees the Universe as dual, as divided

Svapne – in dream; Jāgrati - waking state; Vā – or; Ya – he who; Eṣa – this; Puruṣaḥ - conscious being; Māyā – Illusion; Paribhrāmitaḥ - utterly confused; Tasmai...

Whether dreaming or awake, the thoroughly confused person sees the world and its relationships such as student, teacher, father, son, etc., cloaked in the veil of duality. The Master is one who sees the Universal relationship simply as cause and effect. My deepest salutations to my respected teacher in the form of Dakṣiṇāmūrti.

Verse 9

Bhūram bhāṁsya nalo-nilo – mbaramahar
nātho himāṃśuḥ pumān
Ityābhāti caracara atmakamidaṃ yasyaiva mūrtyaṣṭakam |
Nānyatkiñcana vidyate vimṛśatāṃ yasmāt parasmādvibhoḥ
Tasmai śrīgurumūrtaye nama idaṃ śrīdakṣiṇāmūrtaye ||

Bhūḥ – the earth; Ambhāṁsya – the waters; Analaḥ – fire; Anilaḥ – air; Ambarama – space; Aharnāthaḥ - Sun; Himāṁśuḥ - Moon; Pumān – the individual soul; Iti – verily; Ābhāti – to shine; Cara – moving; Acara – still; Ātmakam – its nature; Idaṁ – this; Yasya – whose; Eva – indeed; Mūrti – form of; Aṣṭakam – Eight fold

Nānyat – nothing else; Kiñcana – there; Vidyate – is; Vimṛśatāṁ - for the student; Yasmāt – from whom; Parasmat – the Supreme Being; Vibhoḥ - who manifests as creation; Tasmai....

Salutations to him whose eight-fold form is comprised of all movable and immovable things and manifests as the five elements, the sun, the moon and the individual soul. For those spiritual seekers who inquire into the true nature of reality, there is nothing other than He who is the supreme lord who manifests himself as the whole of creation. My deepest salutations to my respected teacher in the form of Dakṣiṇāmūrti.

Verse 10

Sarva atmatvam iti sphuṭī kṛtam idaṃ
yasmād amuṣmin stave
Tenāsya śravaṇāt tadartha mananād
dhyānācca saṅkīrtanāt |
Sarva atmatvamahā vibhūti sahitaṃ
syād īśvaratvaṃ svataḥ
Siddhyet tat punar aṣṭadhā pariṇataṃ
caiśvaryam avyāhatam ||

Sarvātmatvam – the state of being the Self of All; Iti – thus; Sphuṭī – clear; Kṛtam – that which is made clear; Idam – this; Yasmāt – because; Amuṣmin – dwelling in this remembrance; Stave – in the song; Tenā – therefore; Asya – of this piece; Śravaṇāt – hearing of this; Tad – that; Artha – meaning; Mananā – from the reflection; Dhyāna – meditating; Saṅkīrtanāt – singing

Sarvātmatvam – of being the Self of All; Mahā – great; Vibhūti – glory; Sahitaṁ - together with; Syādīśvara – the state unity with God; Tvam – you; Svataḥ - as one's own nature; Siddhi – it is accomplished; Ettat – this; Punar – again; Aṣṭadhā – the Eight fold projection; Pariṇatam – transforms; Ca – and; Aiśvaryaṁ – opulence; Avyāhatam – without obstructions;

Thus, from hearing this song, reflecting on its inner meaning and by singing it, the state of "Being the Self of All" is made clear. Further, by the above said methods, one can make this supremely exalted state firmly established within themselves. This will bring about the unobstructed opulence of the Self as well as a clear understanding of creation.

The End

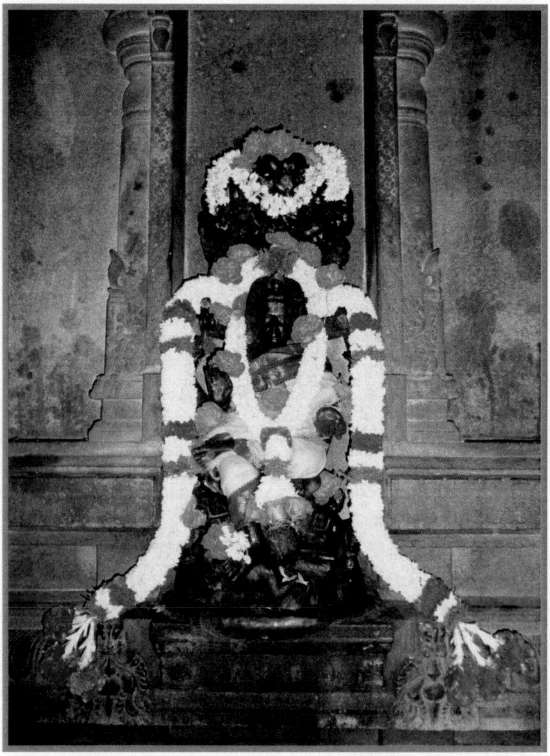

Sunday

30

Revatī			27:11
K 8			10:02
Śobhana			11:10
Kaulava			10:02
Taitila			22:23
Rāhu Kālam	18:42	-	20:32

Monday

1

Aśvinī			29:09
K 9			10:54
Atigaṇḍa			10:54
Gara			10:54
Vanija			23:36
Rāhu Kālam	7:41	-	9:31
Moon: Aries			3:11

Tuesday

2

Bharaṇī			Full Night
K 10			12:26
Sukarmā			11:09
Viṣṭi			12:26
Bava			25:23
Rāhu Kālam	16:52	-	18:42

Wednesday

3

Bharaṇī			7:40
K 11			14:27
Dhṛti			11:47
Bālava			14:27
Kaulava			27:36
Rāhu Kālam	13:12	-	15:02
Moon: Taurus			14:21

Thursday

4

Kṛttikā		10:32	
K 12		16:48	
Śūla		12:41	
Taitila		16:48	
Gara		Full Night	
Rāhu Kālam	15:02	- 16:52	
Mars: Gemini		12:42	Independence Day

Friday

5

Rohinī		13:35	
K 13		19:18	
Gaṇḍa		13:43	
Gara		6:02	
Vanija		19:18	
Rāhu Kālam	11:22	- 13:12	

Saturday

6

Mṛgaśīrṣa		16:40	
K 14		21:49	
Vṛddhi		14:47	
Viṣṭi		8:34	
Śakuni		21:49	
Rāhu Kālam	9:33	- 11:22	
Moon: Gemini		3:07	Birthday of HH Dalai Lama

June 2013

S	M	T	W	T	F	S
						1
2	3	4	5	6	7	8
9	10	11	12	13	14	15
16	17	18	19	20	21	22
23	24	25	26	27	28	29
30						

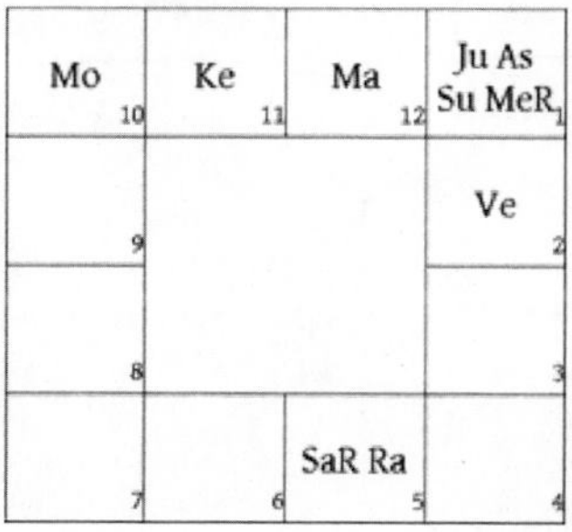

July 2013

S	M	T	W	T	F	S
	1	2	3	4	5	6
7	8	9	10	11	12	13
14	15	16	17	18	19	20
21	22	23	24	25	26	27
28	29	30	31			

Sunday ●

7

Ārdrā			19:41
Āmāvasyā			24:14
Dhruva			15:48
Catuṣpada			11:02
Nāga			24:14
Rāhu Kālam	18:41	-	20:31

Monday

8

Punarvasu			22:32
Ś 1			26:28
Vyāghāta			16:42
Kiṃsthughna			13:23
Bava			26:28
Rāhu Kālam	7:44	-	9:33
Moon: Cancer			15:51

Tuesday

9

Puṣyā			25:10
Ś 2			28:28
Harṣaṇa			17:26
Bālava			15:30
Kaulava			28:28
Rāhu Kālam	16:51	-	18:41

Wednesday

10

Āśleṣā			27:32
Ś 3			Full Night
Vajra			17:57
Taitila			17:22
Gara			Full Night
Rāhu Kālam	13:13	-	15:02

Thursday

11

Maghā		29:32
Ś 3		6:11
Siddhi		18:13
Gara		6:11
Vanijja		18:54
Rāhu Kālam	15:02	- 16:51
Moon: Leo		3:32

Friday

12

Pūrva Phalguṇī		Full Night
Ś 4		7:31
Vyatīpāta		18:10
Viṣṭi		7:31
Bava		20:02
Rāhu Kālam	11:24	- 13:13

Saturday

13

Pūrva Phalguṇī		7:08
Ś 5		8:25
Varīyān		17:46
Bālava		8:25
Kaulava		20:41
Rāhu Kālam	9:35	- 11:24
Moon: Virgo		13:27

July 2013

S	M	T	W	T	F	S
	1	2	3	4	5	6
7	8	9	10	11	12	13
14	15	16	17	18	19	20
21	22	23	24	25	26	27
28	29	30	31			

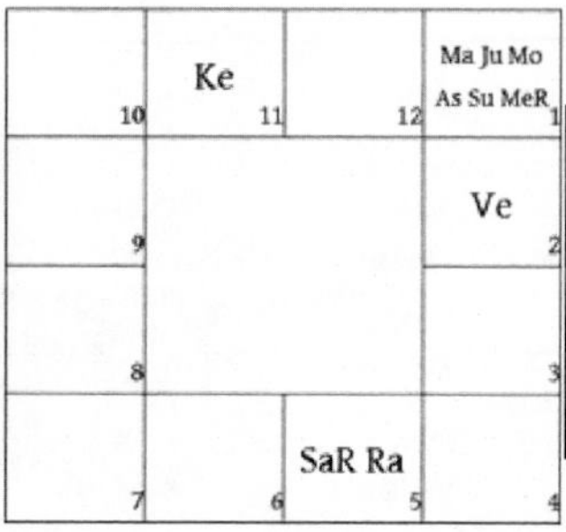

August 2013

S	M	T	W	T	F	S
				1	2	3
4	5	6	7	8	9	10
11	12	13	14	15	16	17
18	19	20	21	22	23	24
25	26	27	28	29	30	31

Sunday
14

Uttara Phalguṇī		8:14	
Ś 6		8:49	
Parigha		16:56	
Taitila		8:49	
Gara		20:48	
Rāhu Kālam	18:39	- 20:28	

Monday
15

Hasta		8:45	
Ś 7		8:38	
Śiva		15:37	
Vanija		8:38	
Viṣṭi		20:18	
Rāhu Kālam	7:48	- 9:36	
Moon: Libra		0:55	

Tuesday
16

Citrā		8:39	
Ś 8		7:48	
Siddha		13:47	
Bava		7:48	
Bālava		19:09	
Rāhu Kālam	16:50	- 18:39	
Sun: Cancer		3:10	Puṇya Kāla: 13:13 - 20:27

Wednesday
17

Svāti		7:54	
Ś 9		6:19	
Ś 10		28:12	
Sādhya		11:26	
Kaulava		6:19	
Taitila		17:20	
Gara		28:12	
Rāhu Kālam	13:13	- 15:02	
Venus: Leo		7:03	

Thursday
18

Viśākhā			6:31
Anurādha			28:34
Ś 11			25:30
Śubha			8:33
Śukla			29:12
Vanijja			18:54
Viṣṭi			25:30
Rāhu Kālam	15:02	-	16:50
Moon: Scorpio			0:55

Friday
19

Jyeṣṭhā			26:07
Ś 12			22:19
Brahma			25:28
Bava			11:57
Bālava			22:19
Rāhu Kālam	11:26	-	13:14

Saturday
20

Mūla			23:22
Ś 13			18:46
Mahendra			21:27
Kaulava			8:34
Taitila			18:46
Gara			28:54
Rāhu Kālam	9:38	-	11:26
Moon: Sagittarius			2:07

July 2013

S	M	T	W	T	F	S
	1	2	3	4	5	6
7	8	9	10	11	12	13
14	15	16	17	18	19	20
21	22	23	24	25	26	27
28	29	30	31			

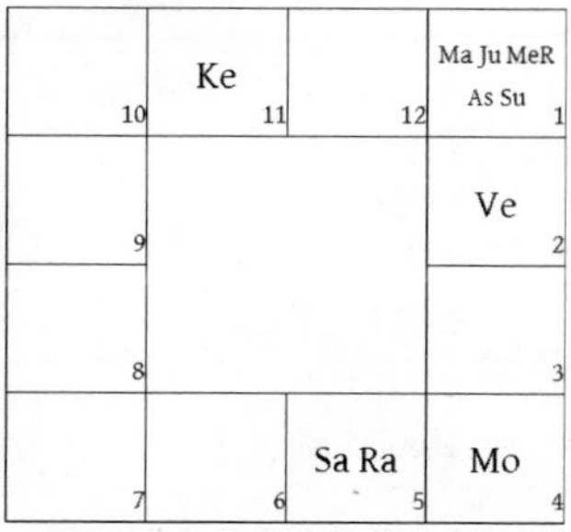

August 2013

S	M	T	W	T	F	S
				1	2	3
4	5	6	7	8	9	10
11	12	13	14	15	16	17
18	19	20	21	22	23	24
25	26	27	28	29	30	31

Sunday
21

Pūrvāṣāḍhā		20:26	
Ś 14		15:01	
Vaidhṛti		17:16	
Vanija		15:01	
Viṣṭi		25:08	
Rāhu Kālam	18:36	- 20:24	

Monday ○
22

Uttarāṣāḍhā		17:31	
Pūrṇimā		11:15	
Viṣkambha		13:06	
Bava		11:15	
Bālava		21:25	
Rāhu Kālam	7:52	- 9:39	
Moon: Capricorn		1:41	Guru Pūrṇimā

Tuesday
23

Śravaṇa		14:49	
K 1		7:38	
K 2		28:21	
Prīti		9:04	
Āyuṣman		29:20	
Kaulava		7:38	
Taitila		17:57	
Gara		28:21	
Rāhu Kālam	16:48	- 18:35	

Wednesday
24

Dhaniṣṭhā		12:32	
K 3		25:36	
Saubhāgya		26:02	
Vanija		14:54	
Viṣṭi		25:36	
Rāhu Kālam	13:14	- 15:01	
Moon: Aquarius		1:37	

Thursday

25

Śatabhiṣā		10:50
K 4		23:30
Śobhana		23:18
Bava		12:28
Bālava		23:30
Rāhu Kālam	15:00	- 16:47

Friday

26

Pūrva Bhādrapadā		9:51
K 5		22:13
Atigaṇḍa		21:12
Kaulava		10:45
Taitila		22:13
Rāhu Kālam	11:27	- 13:14
Moon: Pisces		4:01

Saturday

27

Uttara Bhādrapadā		9:42
K 6		21:47
Sukarmā		19:48
Gara		9:53
Vanija		21:47
Rāhu Kālam	9:41	- 11:27

July 2013

S	M	T	W	T	F	S
	1	2	3	4	5	6
7	8	9	10	11	12	13
14	15	16	17	18	19	20
21	22	23	24	25	26	27
28	29	30	31			

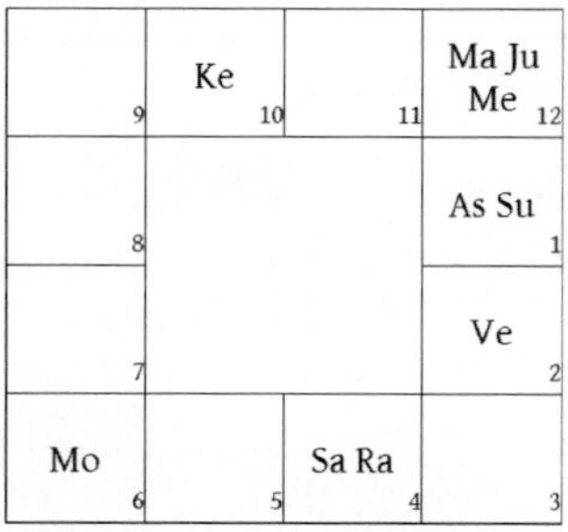

August 2013

S	M	T	W	T	F	S
				1	2	3
4	5	6	7	8	9	10
11	12	13	14	15	16	17
18	19	20	21	22	23	24
25	26	27	28	29	30	31

Sunday

28

Revatī			10:24	
K 7			22:12	
Dhṛti			19:05	
Viṣṭi			9:53	
Bava			22:12	
Rāhu Kālam	18:32	-	20:19	
Moon: Aries			10:24	Parent's Day

Monday

29

Aśvinī			11:55
K 8			23:25
Śūla			18:59
Bālava			10:43
Kaulava			23:25
Rāhu Kālam	7:56	-	9:42

Tuesday

30

Bharaṇī			14:08
K 9			25:15
Gaṇḍa			19:24
Taitila			12:16
Gara			25:15
Rāhu Kālam	16:45	-	18:31
Moon: Taurus			20:46

Wednesday

31

Kṛttikā			16:50
K 10			27:32
Vṛddhi			20:12
Vanija			14:21
Viṣṭi			27:32
Rāhu Kālam	13:14	-	14:59

Thursday

1

Rohinī		19:50
K 11		30:02
Dhruva		21:12
Bava		16:46
Bālava		30:02
Rāhu Kālam	15:00 -	16:47

Lammas • Lughnassad

Friday

2

Mṛgaśīrṣa		22:56
K 12		Full Night
Vyāghāta		22:16
Kaulava		19:18
Taitila		Full Night
Rāhu Kālam	11:28 -	13:13
Moon: Gemini		9:23

Saturday

3

Ārdrā		25:56
K 12		8:33
Harṣaṇa		23:15
Taitila		8:33
Gara		21:46
Rāhu Kālam	9:44 -	11:28

July 2013

S	M	T	W	T	F	S
	1	2	3	4	5	6
7	8	9	10	11	12	13
14	15	16	17	18	19	20
21	22	23	24	25	26	27
28	29	30	31			

Mo 9	Ke 10	11	Ju Ma Me 12
8			As Su 1
7			Ve 2
6	5	Sa Ra 4	3

August 2013

S	M	T	W	T	F	S
				1	2	3
4	5	6	7	8	9	10
11	12	13	14	15	16	17
18	19	20	21	22	23	24
25	26	27	28	29	30	31

Sunday

4

Punarvasu			28:43
K 13			10:56
Vajra			24:05
Vanija			10:56
Viṣṭi			24:01
Rāhu Kālam	18:27	-	20:11
Moon: Cancer			22:03
Mercury: Cancer			9:08

Monday

5

Puṣyā			Full Night
K 14			13:03
Siddhi			24:41
Śakuni			13:03
Catuṣpada			25:59
Rāhu Kālam	8:00	-	9:44

Tuesday ●

6

Puṣyā			7:13
Āmāvasyā			14:50
Vyatīpāta			25:01
Nāga			14:50
Kiṃsthughna			27:36
Rāhu Kālam	16:41	-	18:25

Wednesday

7

Āśleṣā			9:22
Ś 1			16:17
Varīyān			25:05
Bava			16:17
Bālava			28:52
Rāhu Kālam	13:13	-	14:57
Moon: Leo			9:22

Thursday

8

Maghā		11:11
Ś 2		17:21
Parigha		24:52
Kaulava		17:21
Taitila		29:45
Rāhu Kālam	14:56 -	16:40

Eid Ul - Fitr

Friday

9

Pūrva Phalguṇī		12:37
Ś 3		18:03
Śiva		24:12
Gara		18:03
Vanija		30:16
Rāhu Kālam	11:29 -	13:13
Moon: Virgo		18:56

Saturday

10

Uttara Phalguṇī		13:41
Ś 4		18:22
Siddha		23:31
Viṣṭi		18:22
Bava		Full Night
Rāhu Kālam	9:46 -	11:29

August 2013

S	M	T	W	T	F	S
				1	2	3
4	5	6	7	8	9	10
11	12	13	14	15	16	17
18	19	20	21	22	23	24
25	26	27	28	29	30	31

9	Ke 10	11	Ju Ma Mo Me 12
8			As Su 1
7			Ve 2
6	5	Sa Ra 4	3

September 2013

S	M	T	W	T	F	S
1	2	3	4	5	6	7
8	9	10	11	12	13	14
15	16	17	18	19	20	21
22	23	24	25	26	27	28
29	30					

Sunday
11

Hasta			14:21
Ś 5			18:15
Sādhya			22:20
Bava			6:22
Bālava			18:15
Kaulava			30:02
Rāhu Kālam	18:21	-	20:04
Venus: Virgo			8:18

Monday
12

Citrā			14:34
Ś 6			17:41
Śubha			20:48
Taitila			17:41
Gara			29:14
Rāhu Kālam	8:04	-	9:47
Moon: Libra			2:31

Tuesday
13

Svāti			14:19
Ś 7			16:38
Śukla			18:52
Vanija			16:38
Viṣṭi			27:56
Rāhu Kālam	16:36	-	18:19

Wednesday
14

Viśākhā			13:33
Ś 8			15:05
Brahma			16:31
Bava			15:05
Bālava			26:07
Rāhu Kālam	13:12	-	14:54
Moon: Scorpio			7:48

Thursday
15

Anurādha			12:!8	
Ś 9			13:02	
Mahendra			13:46	
Kaulava			13:02	
Taitila			23:50	
Rāhu Kālam	14:53	-	16:35	Assumption Day

Friday
16

Jyeṣṭhā			10:35	
Ś 10			10:31	
Vaidhṛti			10:39	
Gara			10:31	
Vanija			21:07	
Rāhu Kālam	11:30	-	13:11	
Moon: Sagittarius			10:35	
Sun: Leo			11:32	Puṇya Kāla: 4:19 - 11:32

Saturday
17

Mūla			8:30
Pūrvāṣāḍhā			30:07
Ś 11			7:38
Ś 12			28:28
Viṣkambha			7:13
Prīti			27:32
Viṣṭi			7:38
Bava			18:04
Bālava			28:28
Rāhu Kālam	9:49	-	11:30

August 2013

S	M	T	W	T	F	S
				1	2	3
4	5	6	7	8	9	10
11	12	13	14	15	16	17
18	19	20	21	22	23	24
25	26	27	28	29	30	31

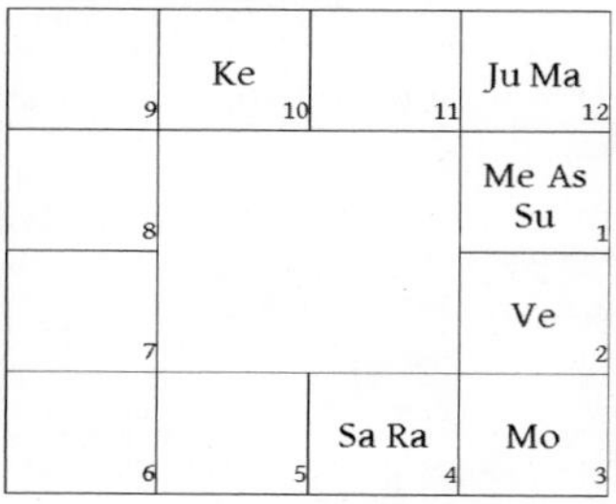

September 2013

S	M	T	W	T	F	S
1	2	3	4	5	6	7
8	9	10	11	12	13	14
15	16	17	18	19	20	21
22	23	24	25	26	27	28
29	30					

Sunday
18

Uttarāṣāḍhā		27:37	
Ś 13		25:09	
Āyuṣman		23:44	
Kaulava		14:49	
Taitila		25:09	
Rāhu Kālam	18:14	- 19:55	
Moon: Capricorn		11:30	
Mars: Cancer		13:29	

Monday
19

Śravaṇa		25:09	
Ś 14		21:51	
Saubhāgya		19:56	
Gara		11:30	
Vanija		21:51	
Rāhu Kālam	8:09	- 9:49	Onam

Tuesday ○
20

Dhaniṣṭhā		22:53	
Pūrṇimā		18:44	
Śobhaṇa		16:16	
Viṣṭi		8:16	
Bava		18:44	
Bālava		29:18	
Rāhu Kālam	16:31	- 18:12	
Moon: Aquarius		11:59	
Mercury: Leo		16:25	Rakṣa Bandhana

Wednesday
21

Śatabhiṣā		21:00	
K 1		15:58	
Atigaṇḍa		12:53	
Kaulava		15:58	
Taitila		26:46	
Rāhu Kālam	13:10	- 14:50	

Thursday

22

Pūrva Bhādrapadā			19:41
K 2			13:42
Sukarmā			9:54
Gara			13:42
Vanija			24:49
Rāhu Kālam	14:50	-	16:30
Moon: Pisces			13:57

Friday

23

Uttara Bhādrapadā			19:02
K 3			12:07
Dhṛti			7:26
Śūla			29:34
Viṣṭi			12:07
Bava			23:36
Rāhu Kālam	11:30	-	13:10

Saturday

24

Revatī			19:10
K 4			11:17
Gaṇḍa			28:21
Bālava			11:17
Kaulava			23:10
Rāhu Kālam	9:51	-	11:30
Moon: Aries			19:10

August 2013

S	M	T	W	T	F	S
				1	2	3
4	5	6	7	8	9	10
11	12	13	14	15	16	17
18	19	20	21	22	23	24
25	26	27	28	29	30	31

8	Ke 9	10	Ju Ma 11
7			Me 12
6			Su As 1
Mo 5	4	Sa Ra 3	Ve 2

September 2013

S	M	T	W	T	F	S
1	2	3	4	5	6	7
8	9	10	11	12	13	14
15	16	17	18	19	20	21
22	23	24	25	26	27	28
29	30					

Sunday
25

Āśvinī			20:07
K 5			11:16
Vṛddhi			27:47
Taitila			11:16
Gara			23:35
Rāhu Kālam	18:06	-	19:45

Monday
26

Bharaṇī			21:50
K 6			12:04
Dhruva			27:48
Vanija			12:04
Viṣṭi			24:45
Rāhu Kālam	8:13	-	9:51

Tuesday
27

Kṛttikā			24:11
K 7			13:36
Vyāghāta			28:18
Bava			13:36
Bālava			26:34
Rāhu Kālam	16:25	-	18:04
Moon: Taurus			4:22

Wednesday
28

Started period

Rohinī			26:58
K 8			15:40
Harṣaṇa			29:08
Kaulava			15:40
Taitila			28:50
Rāhu Kālam	13:08	-	14:46

Śrī Kṛṣṇa Janmāṣṭamī

Thursday

29

Mṛgaśīrṣa			29:59
K 9			18:04
Vajra			30:06
Gara			18:04
Vanija			Full Night
Rāhu Kālam	14:46	-	16:24
Moon: Gemini			16:28

Friday

30

Ārdrā			Full Night
K 10			20:34
Siddhi			Full Night
Vanija			7:19
Viṣṭi			20:34
Rāhu Kālam	11:30	-	13:08

Saturday

31

Ārdrā			8:59
K 11			22:56
Siddhi			7:04
Bava			9:46
Bālava			22:56
Rāhu Kālam	9:53	-	11:30

August 2013

S	M	T	W	T	F	S
				1	2	3
4	5	6	7	8	9	10
11	12	13	14	15	16	17
18	19	20	21	22	23	24
25	26	27	28	29	30	31

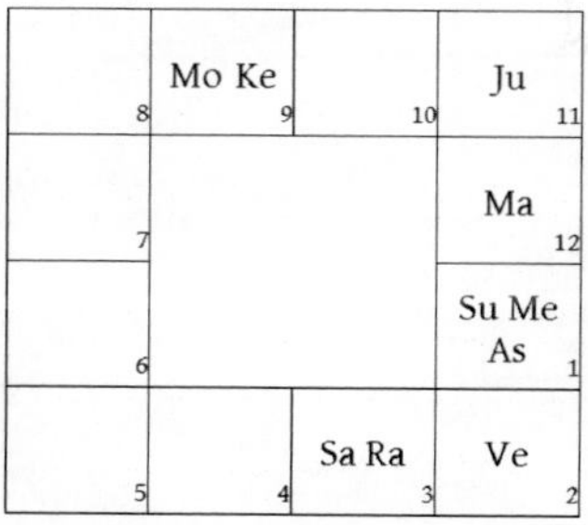

September 2013

S	M	T	W	T	F	S
1	2	3	4	5	6	7
8	9	10	11	12	13	14
15	16	17	18	19	20	21
22	23	24	25	26	27	28
29	30					

Sunday

1

Punarvasu		11:47	
K 12		25:00	
Vyatīpāta		7:53	
Kaulava		12:00	
Taitila		25:00	
Rāhu Kālam	17:58 -	19:35	
Moon: Cancer		5:06	

Monday

2

Puṣyā		14:13	
K 13		26:39	
Varīyān		8:26	
Gara		13:53	
Vanija		26:39	
Rāhu Kālam	8:16 -	9:53	Labor Day

Tuesday

3

Āśleṣā		16:15	
K 14		27:51	
Parigha		8:39	
Viṣṭi		15:19	
Śakuni		27:51	
Rāhu Kālam	16:19 -	17:56	
Moon: Leo		16:15	

Wednesday ●

4

Maghā		17:49	
Āmāvasyā		28:36	
Śiva		8:31	
Catuṣpada		16:17	
Nāga		28:36	
Rāhu Kālam	13:06 -	14:42	Rosh Hashanah

Thursday

5

Pūrva Phalguṇī 18:57
Ś 1 28:53
Siddha 8:01
Kiṃsthughna 16:48
Bava 28:53
Rāhu Kālam 14:41 - 16:17
Mercury: Virgo 16:25
Venus: Libra 20:10

Friday

6

Uttara Phalguṇī 19:40
Ś 2 28:47
Sādhya 7:10
Śubha 30:01
Bālava 16:53
Kaulava 28:47
Rāhu Kālam 11:30 - 13:05
Moon: Virgo 1:10

Saturday

7

Hasta 20:00
Ś 3 28:18
Śukla 28:34
Taitila 16:35
Gara 28:18
Rāhu Kālam 9:54 - 11:30

September 2013

S	M	T	W	T	F	S
1	2	3	4	5	6	7
8	9	10	11	12	13	14
15	16	17	18	19	20	21
22	23	24	25	26	27	28
29	30					

8	Ke 9	10	Ju 11
7			Mo Ma 12
6			Su As Me 1
5	4	Sa Ra 3	Ve 2

October 2013

S	M	T	W	T	F	S
		1	2	3	4	5
6	7	8	9	10	11	12
13	14	15	16	17	18	19
20	21	22	23	24	25	26
27	28	29	30	31		

Sunday
8

Citrā			20:00	
Ś 4			27:29	
Brahma			26:50	
Vanija			15:56	
Viṣṭi			27:29	
Rāhu Kālam	17:49	-	19:24	
Moon: Libra			8:03	Gaṇeśa Caturthī

Monday
9

Svāti			19:41	
Ś 5			26:21	
Mahendra			24:51	
Bava			14:57	
Bālava			26:21	
Rāhu Kālam	8:20	-	9:55	

Tuesday
10

Viśākhā			19:02	
Ś 6			24:53	
Vaidhṛti			22:37	
Kaulava			13:39	
Taitila			24:53	
Rāhu Kālam	16:13	-	17:47	
Moon: Scorpio			13:13	

Wednesday
11

Anurādha			18:05	
Ś 7			23:07	
Viṣkambha			20:07	
Gara			12:02	
Vanija			23:07	
Rāhu Kālam	13:04	-	14:38	Patriot Day

Thursday
12

Jyeṣṭhā			16:51	
Ś 8			21:04	
Prīti			17:24	
Viṣṭi			10:08	
Bava			21:04	
Rāhu Kālam	14:37	-	16:11	
Moon: Sagittarius			16:51	

Friday
13

Mūla			15:21	
Ś 9			18:46	
Āyuṣman			14:27	
Bālava			7:57	
Kaulava			18:46	
Taitila			29:32	
Rāhu Kālam	11:29	-	13:03	Yom Kippur starts

Saturday
14

Pūrvāṣāḍhā			13:38	
Ś 10			16:16	
Saubhāgya			11:20	
Gara			16:16	
Vanija			26:58	
Rāhu Kālam	9:56	-	11:29	
Moon: Capricorn			19:11	Yom Kippur ends

September 2013

S	M	T	W	T	F	S
1	2	3	4	5	6	7
8	9	10	11	12	13	14
15	16	17	18	19	20	21
22	23	24	25	26	27	28
29	30					

8	Ke 9	10	Ju 11
7			Ma 12
6			As Su 1
5	4	Ve Sa Ra 3	Me Mo 2

October 2013

S	M	T	W	T	F	S
		1	2	3	4	5
6	7	8	9	10	11	12
13	14	15	16	17	18	19
20	21	22	23	24	25	26
27	28	29	30	31		

Sunday
15

Uttarāṣāḍhā			11:48	
Ś 11			13:39	
Śobhana			8:07	
Atigaṇḍa			28:50	
Viṣṭi			13:39	
Bava			24:19	
Rāhu Kālam	17:41	-	19:14	

Monday
16

Śravaṇa			9:56	
Ś 12			11:00	
Sukarmā			25:37	
Bālava			11:00	
Kaulava			21:43	
Rāhu Kālam	8:24	-	9:57	
Moon: Aquarius			21:01	
Sun: Virgo			11:28	Puṇya Kāla: 11:28 - 18:10

Tuesday
17

Dhaniṣṭhā			8:09	
Śatabhiṣā			30:36	
Ś 13			8:28	
Ś 14			30:09	
Dhṛti			22:33	
Taitila			8:28	
Gara			19:16	
Vanija			30:09	
Rāhu Kālam	16:06	-	17:38	

Wednesday ○
18

Pūrva Bhādrapadā			29:25	
Pūrṇimā			28:12	
Śūla			19:45	
Viṣṭi			17:08	
Bava			28:12	
Rāhu Kālam	13:01	-	14:33	
Moon: Pisces			23:40	Sukkot

Thursday

19

Uttara Bhādrapadā		28:44	
K 1		26:45	
Gaṇḍa		17:18	
Bālava		15:25	
Kaulava		26:45	
Rāhu Kālam	14:32 -	16:04	Pitṛ Pakṣa Starts (Śrāddha)

Friday

20

Revatī		28:39	
K 2		25:55	
Vṛddhi		15:18	
Taitila		14:15	
Gara		25:55	
Rāhu Kālam	11:29 -	13:00	

Saturday

21

Aśvinī		29:15	
K 3		25:45	
Dhruva		13:50	
Vanija		13:45	
Viṣṭi		25:45	
Rāhu Kālam	9:58 -	11:29	
Moon: Aries		4:39	International Peace Day

September 2013

S	M	T	W	T	F	S
1	2	3	4	5	6	7
8	9	10	11	12	13	14
15	16	17	18	19	20	21
22	23	24	25	26	27	28
29	30					

8	Ke 9	10	Ju 11
7			Ma 12
Mo 6			As Su 1
5	4	Ve Sa Ra 3	Me 2

October 2013

S	M	T	W	T	F	S
		1	2	3	4	5
6	7	8	9	10	11	12
13	14	15	16	17	18	19
20	21	22	23	24	25	26
27	28	29	30	31		

Sunday

22

Bharaṇī			30:33	
K 4			26:20	
Vyāghāta			12:55	
Bava			13:57	
Bālava			26:20	
Rāhu Kālam	17:32	-	19:03	Mabon • Autumnal Equinox 13:44

Monday

23

Kṛttikā			Full Night
K 5			27:35
Harṣaṇa			12:34
Kaulava			14:52
Taitila			27:35
Rāhu Kālam	8:28	-	9:58
Moon: Taurus			12:59

Tuesday

Started period

24

Kṛttikā			8:30
K 6			29:26
Vajra			12:43
Gara			16:27
Vanija			29:26
Rāhu Kālam	15:59	-	17:29
Mercury: Libra			18:03

Wednesday

Should start period

25

Rohiṇī			11:00
K 7			Full Night
Siddhi			13:16
Viṣṭi			18:32
Bava			Full Night
Rāhu Kālam	12:59	-	14:29

Thursday

26

Mṛgaśīrṣa			13:51
K 7			7:42
Vyatīpāta			14:05
Bava			7:42
Bālava			20:55
Rāhu Kālam	14:28	-	15:57
Moon: Gemini			0:24

Friday

27

Ārdrā			16:49
K 8			10:09
Varīyān			15:00
Kaulava			10:09
Taitila			23:23
Rāhu Kālam	11:29	-	12:58

Amma's Birthday • Native American's Day

Saturday

28

Punarvasu			19:42
K 9			12:34
Parigha			15:51
Gara			12:34
Vanija			25:41
Rāhu Kālam	10:00	-	11:29
Moon: Cancer			13:00

September 2013

S	M	T	W	T	F	S
1	2	3	4	5	6	7
8	9	10	11	12	13	14
15	16	17	18	19	20	21
22	23	24	25	26	27	28
29	30					

7	Mo Ke 8	9	Ju 10
6			Ma 11
5			12
4	3	Ra Sa Ve 2	As Su Me 1

October 2013

S	M	T	W	T	F	S
		1	2	3	4	5
6	7	8	9	10	11	12
13	14	15	16	17	18	19
20	21	22	23	24	25	26
27	28	29	30	31		

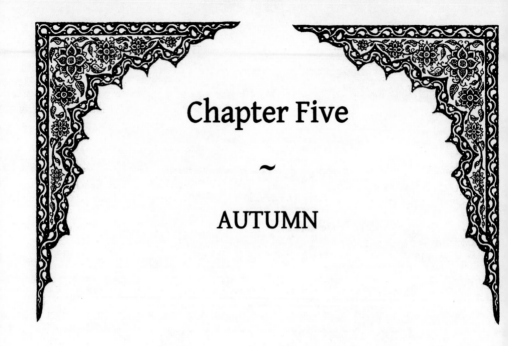

Chapter Five

~

AUTUMN

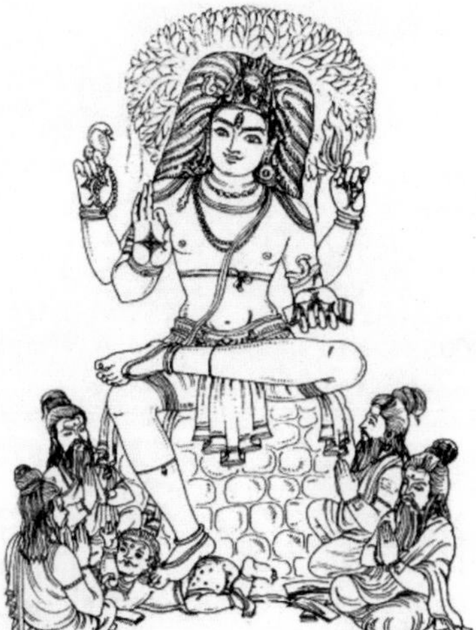

Dakṣiṇāmūrti and the Four Sons of Brahmā

~

Part II

The four brothers were now bound tightly to their noble quest for Truth. First on their pilgrimage, they came to the abode of Lord Viṣṇu, the world known as Vaikuṇṭha. As they approached the palatial doors to Viṣṇu's mansion, they marveled at the sparkling emeralds and other costly gems that were set in them. The entryway was guarded by spotlessly dressed sentries. As the brothers approached, the sentries spoke. "O noble seekers, you have come upon the royal residence of Lord Viṣṇu, the God who is the sole supporter of all of creation; without him, nothing can be sustained. Tell us, what is it that has brought you here?"

"We have come seeking the highest," Sanat Kumāra said. "We wish to have an audience with Lord Viṣṇu so that he may teach us Self Knowledge."

"Very well, please follow me," the head sentry spoke. "Lord Viṣṇu will be delighted to host such earnest seekers. I will take you to his chambers at once."

The brothers passed through various courtyards expertly decorated with all varieties of blooming flowers, chambers where priests were performing grand offering ceremonies and seemingly endless stately rooms used for hosting large banquets. The air inside of the palace was heavily perfumed with various sweet scents. At last, the group arrived at the hall where Lord Viṣṇu was seated. There were highly skilled musicians playing enchanting music, servants standing at the ready for the God's every desire and different Demi-Gods throughout the room engaged in games, joking and revelry. As they entered, they also noticed Viṣṇu's wife standing behind him, massaging him fondly.

"Greetings, wise ones! Welcome to my home. Why is it that I

have been so fortunate as to have been graced by your visit?" Lord Viṣṇu spoke in an authoritative voice.

"Namaste, Your Worshipfulness," the seekers said. "We four are sons of Lord Brahmā and have come on a most important mission. Knowing that you are solely responsible for sustaining the entire creation, we wish to learn from you the essence of spirituality. We wish to be instructed on the Knowledge of the Self."

"Ah, most excellent!" Lord Viṣṇu bellowed. "Most excellent indeed! Yes, I *will* do as you four request but let us not make unnecessary haste. First, I would be delighted for you all to join me as my esteemed guests at the banquet that I am about to host. You are just in time, as the festivities will start tomorrow. First, there will be one year of pre-banquet celebrations, then a grand banquet will commence that will last another year and finally we will conclude with one more extended gala of merriment to celebrate what a fine job we have done."

The four brothers swallowed as they looked at each other hesitantly.

"Won't you join us?" Lord Viṣṇu asked.

"Thank you very much Lord ... but actually ... we really must be getting on our way now. Thank you indeed for the offer, as well as for the hospitality that you have shown us. All the best, goodbye!" they choked out as they were quickly retracing their steps out of the room.

Once they had walked well beyond the palace gates, Sanat Kumāra spoke first, "Oh my goodness, I thought that we were done for!"

"Me too!" Sanaka confirmed.

"What shall we do now?" Sanat Sujāta asked.

"I have an idea," Sānanda spoke, a gleam brightening in his eye. "Our father, Lord Brahmā, is responsible for creating the worlds, while Lord Viṣṇu has his hands full sustaining them. Why we don't inquire at Mount Kailāsa where the Lord of destruction resides? If he spends so much time focused on the dissolution of Reality, he must have a good reason for it? What I mean to say is that he must understand the impermanence of the world if he is so opportune to destroy it. Let us find Lord Śiva, so that we might gain ultimate insight into the knowledge of the Self."

And so it was decided. The four brothers let not another minute pass before starting their journey. With a fresh beat in their step and renewed confidence that they would soon be able to fully understand the Self of all, they continued their epic quest.

Meanwhile, through his omniscience, Lord Śiva came to find out of the approaching sages and their noble intention. He felt the earnestness within their hearts and knew that he alone held the key to unlock their deepest desire. Understanding his duty, Lord Śiva temporarily bid farewell to his wife Umā and sons Gaṇapati and Murugan and went to the lake Mānasarovar, which lies just in the shadow of the mighty Kailāsa. Assuming the form of Dakṣiṇāmūrti, the Lord sat under a banyan tree along the edge of the lake, holding his hand in the benedictory *Cin-mudra.* Here, he waited for the four seekers.

Not long after, the brothers arrived at the bank of the holy Mānasarovar Lake. After a quick dip in its cooling waters so as to refresh themselves for Lord Dakṣiṇāmūrti, the four sages approached the banyan tree that Dakṣiṇāmūrti was seated under. Prostrating themselves fully before the Lord, the sages then arose and with folded palms, circumambulated him three times. Settling at Dakṣiṇāmūrti's feet, an air of deep serenity began to fill the space around the five beings and a profound peace started to grow within the brother's hearts. They knew at once that they had found that Exalted Soul who could ferry them across the ocean of worldly existence. They had found their guru!

They proceeded to ask Lord Dakṣiṇāmūrti shrewd and penetrating questions about the nature of Reality and the means for attaining the Self. The dialogue between the able teacher and fit students went on unabatedly for many days. The love and tenderness that Dakṣiṇāmūrti showed to the brothers for their sincerity flowed continuously. One after the next, Dakṣiṇāmūrti answered each and every one of their poignant questions. The primordial master was deeply pleased to see the wisdom, dispassion and earnestness within his disciples. This session continued on for quite a long time.

After many of the subtle, spiritual subjects had been covered in minute detail, it dawned in Dakṣiṇāmūrti's pure mind that not through words alone, would the brothers would gain the ultimate experience of the Self. Dakṣiṇāmūrti closed his eyes. Resolving his mind into the very essence of the Self of all, Dakṣiṇāmūrti again brought his right hand up into the Cin-mudra. He then allowed his very being to dissolve into the supreme silence of samādhi.

Because of the deep understanding that had further ripened within the four brothers as a result of Dakṣiṇāmūrti teachings, they too now understood that intellectual understanding can only bring a seeker so far. They closed their eyes. Their minds were now like a freshly fallen snow – pure, silent, serene. Without a single thought arising, the only thing left within the brothers was that of a knowingness of the Self. The five souls now sat together in silence, under the shade of the banyan tree, on the pristine banks of the Lake Mānasarovar, within sight of the mighty Mount Kailāsa, in silence. The very essence of each of the brothers had resolved into the Self of all.

This tale is a rendition of the version recounted by the saint of Aruṇācala, Bhagavan Śrī Rāmaṇa Mahārṣi. Curious about why Dakṣiṇāmūrti, who was known for abiding in silence, had spoken at length to the four sagely brothers, one of Rāmaṇa's devotees asked him this very question. Rāmaṇa authoritatively answered, "Never mind *why* he spoke, this is exactly how it actually happened!"

The End

Hasta Sāmudrika Śāstra

~

The Air Hand

As the heat of summer subsides and turns into the coolness of fall, the nights become chill and the air brisk. This is the time when autumn winds scatter seeds far and wide across the earth.

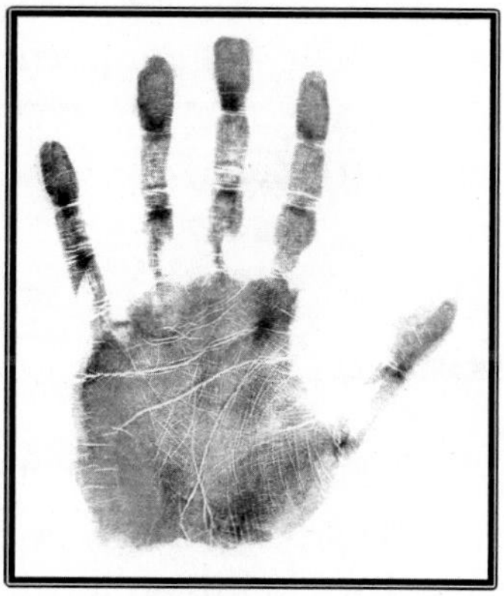

Just as a breeze makes tree leaves dance and carries the fragrance of flowers, those most influenced by the air element live lives that in some way emphasize the art of communication. Essential to communication, air enables the movement, interchange and transmission at the core of the exchange of information and ideas. Those with air hands like to connect things, places and ideas and are typically good at theorizing and conceptualizing. They are thoughtful, friendly, open-minded and supportive of others.

Palm

Air hands have square palms but unlike the rigid square palm of the earth hand, the typical air-hand palm is more flexible and elastic. A square palm indicates solidity and rationality and this mirrors the emotional balance typical of those with air hands.

Air-hand types value the intellect's discriminatory capacity. They are inclined to intellectualize everything and so tend to be especially objective and emotionally centered. As long as their emotions (manifesting as likes and dislikes) are kept in check, they are able to maintain a certain objectivity (and dispassion) in their thoughts and actions. The drawback is that air-handed people can easily live too much in their heads and appear emotionally superficial and cold.

Fingers

An air hand has long fingers which also helps differentiate it from the square-palmed, shorter-fingered earth hand. Long fingers indicate a person with the capacity for great patience and abundant attention to detail. For an air-handed person, the details they collect about the world are organized and categorized in square-palmed fashion and it is this precise, ordered thinking that makes them excellent communicators. They love learning and usually enjoy talking, writing and connecting with others through groups, computers and social networks.

People with air hands truly enjoy finding solutions to complex situations, especially ones that challenge their minds and require them to use their accumulated knowledge. Strategy games and crossword puzzles are a great way to spend some quality time with your air-handed friends.

Skin Texture

The typical air hand has a softness to it, both in its form and in the quality of the skin. Though not as smooth as that of a typical water hand, the skin of an air hand is usually smoother than that of an earth or fire hand. The softness of the air hand reflects the softness of the air-handed person's nature. The air-hand type is rarely contentious about their ideas (that would indicate their emotions are more powerful than their reason). They are often gentle and attracted to a quiet but active life. They typically enjoy living in cities where they have ready access to educational institutions, libraries, theaters and other places that satisfy their thoughtful curiosity. The refinement of their hands makes them suited to a lifestyle where mental activity, as opposed to physical effort, is prevalent.

Lines

The lines of an air hand are typically thin and deep. They look wispy and elegant, as if they have been finely etched into the palm. These lines usually curve and blend into other lines without cutting through them.

How a person perceives their environment is reflected in the line quality of their hands. So, those with air hands have a curious nature and view the world as something to be understood. Yet not all in life is amenable to being categorized and understood especially in the realm of human emotions and interactions and this is one of the lifelong lessons for the air-hand type.

Fingerprints

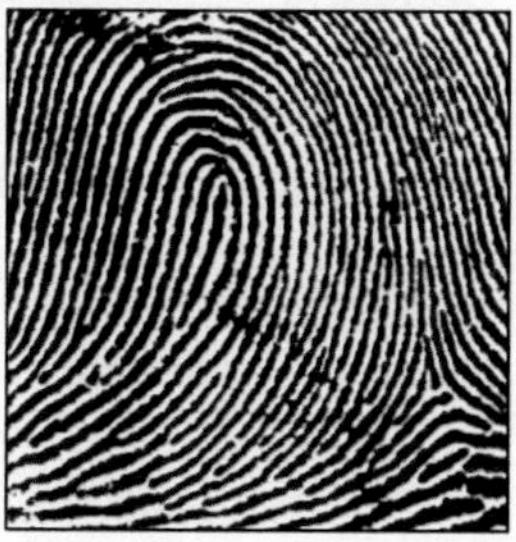

Similar to the water hand, the typical fingerprint pattern for an air hand is the loop. Often the loops on air fingers travel high into the upper part of the digit, which is an added marking for intelligence. Loops indicate gregariousness and an easy-going attitude.

Air-handed folks with multiple loop fingerprints make excellent advisors because they are able to keep an open mind, look at both sides of a situation impartially and keep their emotional reactions to a minimum.

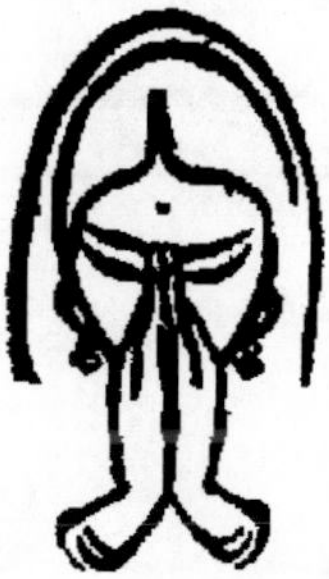

Hasta Sāmudrika Śāstra
~
Which Hand Type are You?

The whole manifest Universe is comprised of the five elements in various permutations. All five elements exist in every person to varying degrees and it is the task of the palmist – the Hasta practitioner – to determine which element prevails in a set of hands. Is it earth, water, fire or air? Determining this is the foundation upon which rich, detailed analysis of lines and markings is built.

As covered in Kālāmṛta's seasonal articles, the structure of the hand is the lead indicator of hand type:

◊ A square palm with short fingers defines an earth hand.

◊ A square palm with long fingers characterizes an air hand.

◊ A rectangular, narrow palm with short fingers shows a fire hand.

◊ A rectangular, narrow palm with long fingers defines a water hand.

Air

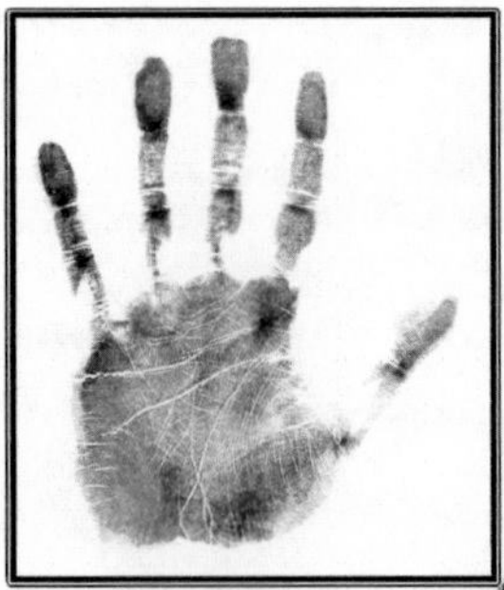

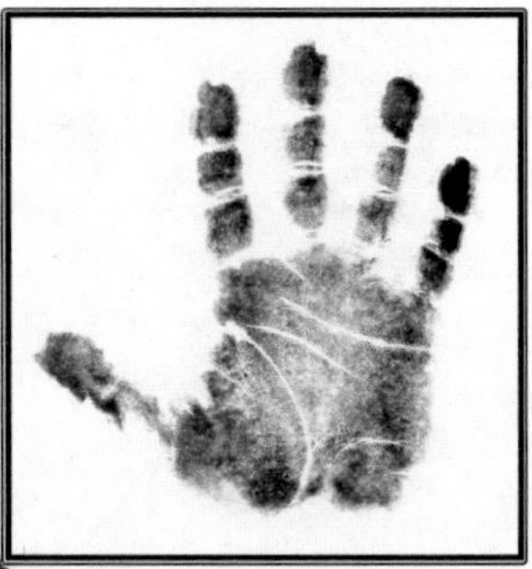

Earth

Fire

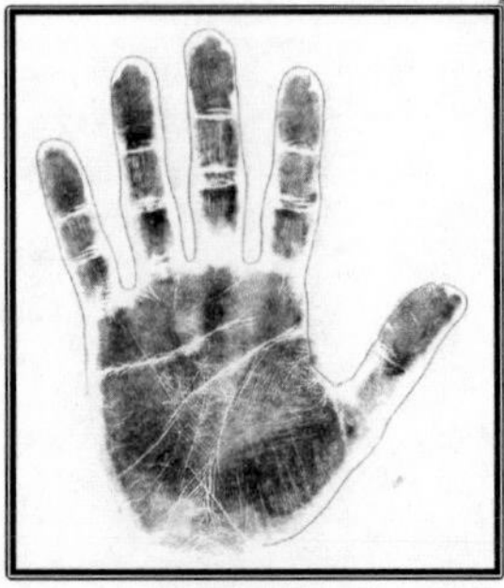

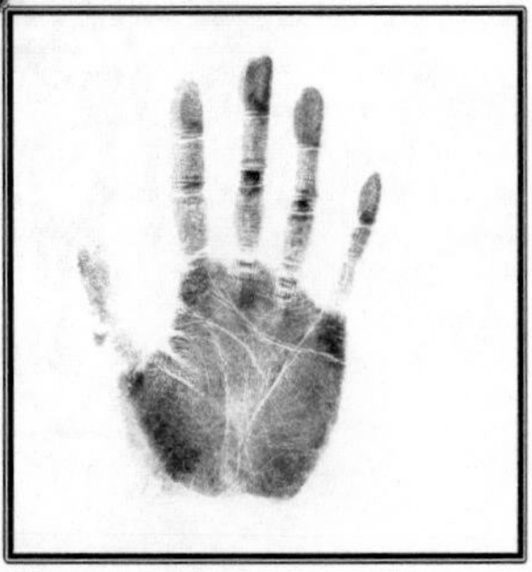

Water

About nine times out of ten, hands will conform to one of these four types. Sometimes though, classifying a hand by its structure is a challenge and so we must recruit other characteristics such as fingerprint pattern and line type to make a determination. For example, let's say that we have a rectangular palm with fingers that are neither short nor long. Is this a water hand or a fire hand? To find the answer, we can look to the fingerprints. Say the set of hands shows eight whorl fingerprints – now the deck is stacked in the direction of these being fire hands because water hands are unlikely to have that many whorls.

Though infrequent, there are also hands that strongly display multiple elements simultaneously. In such cases, we can expect the person to exhibit a wider range of behaviors and greater variety of approaches to life's circumstances.

Ultimately, hand analysis is an elegant dance between the categories presented here and how they uniquely express themselves in a person's life. The most powerful tool we can bring to bear on the subject is a healthy curiosity towards how hands reflect our character and destiny patterns and how they can become a wonderful tool for self-discovery and understanding others and the world around us more intimately.

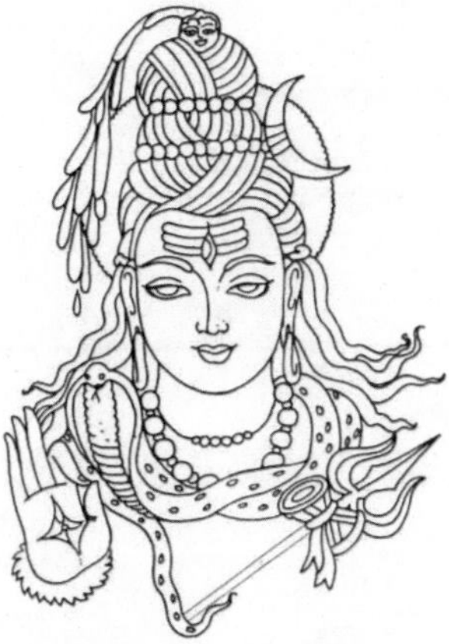

Sunday
29

Puṣyā			22:16
K 10			14:43
Śiva			16:28
Viṣṭi			14:43
Bala			27:38
Rāhu Kālam	17:23	-	18:52

Monday
30

Āśleṣā			24:22
K 11			16:25
Siddha			16:45
Bālava			16:25
Kaulava			29:04
Rāhu Kālam	8:32	-	10:00

Tuesday
1

Maghā			25:56
K 12			17:34
Sādhya			16:37
Taitila			17:34
Gara			29:56
Rāhu Kālam	15:53	-	17:21
Moon: Leo			0:22

Wednesday
2

Pūrva Phalguṇī			26:55
K 13			18:08
Śubha			16:01
Vanija			18:08
Viṣṭi			30:12
Rāhu Kālam	12:56	-	14:24
Venus: Scorpio			2:23

Thursday
3

Uttara Phalguṇī		27:21	
K 14		18:07	
Śukla		14:57	
Śakuni		18:07	
Catuṣpada		29:54	
Rāhu Kālam	14:23	- 15:51	
Moon: Virgo		9:04	

Friday
4

Hasta		27:17	
Āmāvasyā		17:34	
Brahma		13:28	
Nāga		17:34	
Kiṃsthughna		29:07	
Rāhu Kālam	11:29	- 12:56	Pitṛ Pakṣa Ends (Śrāddha)

Saturday
5

Citrā		26:47	
Ś 1		16:33	
Mahendra		11:37	
Bava		16:33	
Bālava		27:54	
Rāhu Kālam	10:02	- 11:29	
Moon: Libra		15:05	
Mars: Leo		7:11	Śārada Navarātrī Begins

September 2013

S	M	T	W	T	F	S
1	2	3	4	5	6	7
8	9	10	11	12	13	14
15	16	17	18	19	20	21
22	23	24	25	26	27	28
29	30					

7	Ke 8	9	Ju 10
6			Mo Ma 11
5			12
4	3	Me Ra Sa Ve 2	As Su 1

October 2013

S	M	T	W	T	F	S
		1	2	3	4	5
6	7	8	9	10	11	12
13	14	15	16	17	18	19
20	21	22	23	24	25	26
27	28	29	30	31		

Sunday

6

Svāti			25:58
Ś 2			15:10
Vaidhṛti			9:26
Viṣkambha			31:00
Kaulava			15:10
Taitila			26:21
Rāhu Kālam	17:15	-	18:41

Monday

7

Viśākhā			24:52
Ś 3			13:28
Prīti			28:21
Gara			13:28
Vanija			24:33
Rāhu Kālam	8:36	-	10:02
Moon: Scorpio			19:10

Tuesday

8

Anurādha			23:36
Ś 4			11:34
Āyuṣman			25:35
Viṣṭi			11:34
Bava			22:33
Rāhu Kālam	15:46	-	17:12

Wednesday

9

Jyeṣṭhā			22:13
Ś 5			9:30
Saubhāgya			22:43
Bālava			9:30
Kaulava			20:26
Rāhu Kālam	12:54	-	14:20
Venus: Sagittarius			22:13

Thursday
10

Mūla			20:45
Ś 6			7:20
Ś 7			29:08
Śobhana			19:47
Taitila			7:20
Gara			18:14
Vanija			29:08
Rāhu Kālam	14:19	-	15:45

Friday
11

Pūrvāṣāḍhā			19:17	
Ś 8			26:56	
Atigaṇḍa			16:51	
Viṣṭi			16:02	
Bava			26:56	
Rāhu Kālam	11:29	-	12:54	Durgā Aṣṭhamī

Saturday
12

Uttarāṣāḍhā			17:51	
Ś 9			24:48	
Sukarmā			13:56	
Bala			13:51	
Kaulava			24:48	
Rāhu Kālam	10:04	-	11:29	
Moon: Capricorn			00:55	Mahā Navamī

October 2013

S	M	T	W	T	F	S
		1	2	3	4	5
6	7	8	9	10	11	12
13	14	15	16	17	18	19
20	21	22	23	24	25	26
27	28	29	30	31		

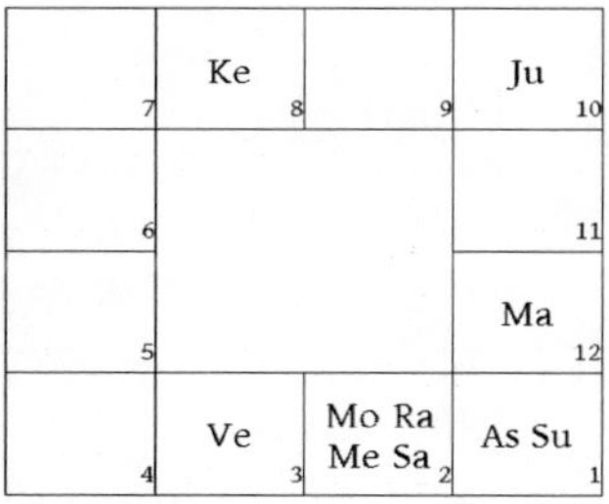

November 2013

S	M	T	W	T	F	S
					1	2
3	4	5	6	7	8	9
10	11	12	13	14	15	16
17	18	19	20	21	22	23
24	25	26	27	28	29	30

Sunday
13

Śravaṇa			16:30	
Ś 10			22:46	
Dhṛti			11:05	
Taitila			11:45	
Gara			22:46	
Rāhu Kālam	17:07	-	18:31	Vijaya Daśamī

Monday
14

Dhaniṣṭhā			15:19	
Ś 11			20:54	
Śūla			8:21	
Gaṇḍa			29:46	
Vanija			9:48	
Viṣṭi			20:54	
Rāhu Kālam	8:41	-	10:05	
Moon: Aquarius			3:53	Columbus Day • Eid al-Adha

Tuesday
15

Śatabhiṣa			14:21	
Ś 12			19:17	
Vṛddhi			27:25	
Bava			8:03	
Bālava			19:17	
Kaulava			30:35	
Rāhu Kālam	15:41	-	17:04	

Wednesday
16

Pūrva Bhādrapadā			13:40	
Ś 13			17:58	
Dhruva			25:19	
Taitila			17:58	
Gara			29:28	
Rāhu Kālam	12:53	-	14:16	
Moon: Pisces			7:48	
Sun: Libra			23:26	Puṇya Kāla: 12:52 - 18:27

Thursday

17

Uttara Bhādrapadā			13:22
Ś 14			17:04
Vyāghāta			23:34
Vanija			17:04
Viṣṭi			28:47
Rāhu Kālam	14:16	-	15:39

Friday ○

18

Revatī			13:30
Pūrṇimā			16:37
Harṣaṇa			22:11
Bava			16:37
Bālava			28:36
Rāhu Kālam	11:29	-	12:52
Moon: Aries			13:30

Saturday

19

Aśvinī			14:09
K 1			16:42
Vajra			21:14
Kaulava			16:42
Taitila			28:58
Rāhu Kālam	10:07	-	11:29

Sweetest Day

October 2013

S	M	T	W	T	F	S
		1	2	3	4	5
6	7	8	9	10	11	12
13	14	15	16	17	18	19
20	21	22	23	24	25	26
27	28	29	30	31		

7	Ke 8	9	Ju 10
6			11
Mo 5			Ma 12
4	Ve 3	Ra Sa Me 2	As Su 1

November 2013

S	M	T	W	T	F	S
					1	2
3	4	5	6	7	8	9
10	11	12	13	14	15	16
17	18	19	20	21	22	23
24	25	26	27	28	29	30

Sunday

20

Bharaṇī		15:21
K 2		17:22
Siddhi		20:44
Gara		17:22
Vanija		29:55
Rāhu Kālam	16:59 -	18:22
Moon: Taurus		21:44

Monday

21

Kṛttikā		17:06
K 3		18:36
Vyatīpāta		20:39
Viṣṭi		18:36
Bava		Full Night
Rāhu Kālam	8:45 -	10:07

Tuesday

Started period

22

Rohinī		19:22
K 4		20:21
Varīyān		20:58
Bava		7:25
Bālava		20:21
Rāhu Kālam	15:35 -	16:57

Wednesday

~~Should start period~~

23

Mṛgaśīrṣa		22:02
K 5		22:32
Parigha		21:36
Kaulava		9:24
Taitila		22:32
Rāhu Kālam	12:51 -	14:13
Moon: Gemini		8:39

Thursday

24

Ārdrā			24:57
K 6			24:59
Śiva			22:25
Gara			11:44
Vanija			24:59
Rāhu Kālam	14:13	-	15:34

Friday

25

Punarvasu			27:54
K 7			27:28
Siddha			23:18
Viṣṭi			14:14
Bava			27:28
Rāhu Kālam	11:30	-	12:51
Moon: Cancer			21:10

Saturday

26

Puṣyā			30:42
K 8			29:47
Sādhya			24:05
Bālava			16:40
Kaulava			29:47
Rāhu Kālam	10:10	-	11:30

October 2013

S	M	T	W	T	F	S
		1	2	3	4	5
6	7	8	9	10	11	12
13	14	15	16	17	18	19
20	21	22	23	24	25	26
27	28	29	30	31		

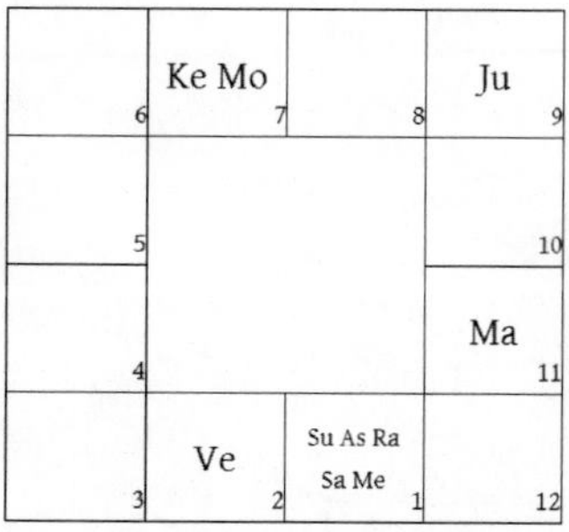

November 2013

S	M	T	W	T	F	S
					1	2
3	4	5	6	7	8	9
10	11	12	13	14	15	16
17	18	19	20	21	22	23
24	25	26	27	28	29	30

Sunday
27

Āśleṣā			Full Night
K 9			Full Night
Śubha			24:36
Taitila			18:49
Gara			Full Night
Rāhu Kālam	16:52	-	18:13

Monday
28

Āśleṣā			9:07
K 9			7:43
Śukla			24:43
Gara			7:43
Vanija			20:29
Rāhu Kālam	8:50	-	10:11
Moon: Leo			9:07

Tuesday
29

Maghā			10:59
K 10			9:06
Brahma			24:21
Viṣṭi			9:06
Bava			21:32
Rāhu Kālam	15:31	-	16:51

Wednesday
30

Pūrva Phalguṇī			12:12
K 11			9:48
Mahendra			23:26
Bālava			9:48
Kaulava			21:52
Rāhu Kālam	12:51	-	14:10
Moon: Virgo			18:24
Venus: Sagittarius			1:54

Thursday

31

Uttara Phalguṇī 12:44
K 12 9:47
Vaidhṛti 21:57
Taitila 9:47
Gara 21:30
Rāhu Kālam 14:10 - 15:30 Halloween • Samain

Friday

1

Hasta 12:34
K 13 9:04
Viṣkambha 19:57
Vanija 9:04
Viṣṭi 20:28
Rāhu Kālam 11:32 - 12:51 All Saints Day

Saturday

2

Citrā 11:49
K 14 7:43
Āmāvasyā 28:49
Śakuni 7:43
Catuṣpada 18:50
Nāga 28:49
Rāhu Kālam 10:13 - 11:32
Moon: Libra 00:16 All Souls Day • Dīwalī

October 2013

S	M	T	W	T	F	S
		1	2	3	4	5
6	7	8	9	10	11	12
13	14	15	16	17	18	19
20	21	22	23	24	25	26
27	28	29	30	31		

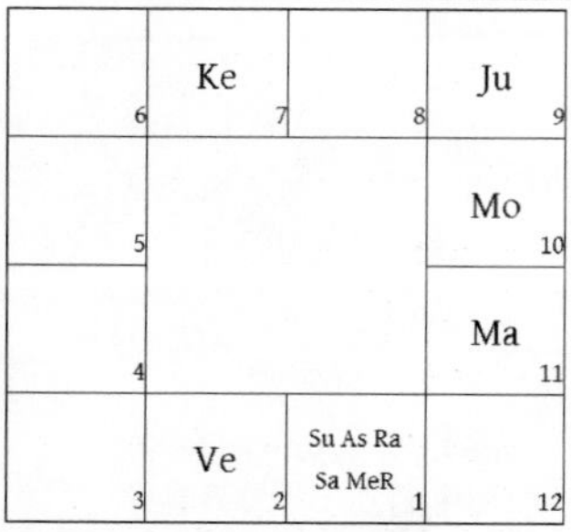

November 2013

S	M	T	W	T	F	S
					1	2
3	4	5	6	7	8	9
10	11	12	13	14	15	16
17	18	19	20	21	22	23
24	25	26	27	28	29	30

Sunday
3

Svāti			9:32	
Ś 1			26:31	
Āyuṣman			13:37	
Kiṃsthughna			15:43	
Bava			26:31	
Rāhu Kālam	15:46	-	17:05	Daylight Savings ends

Monday
4

Viśākhā			7:53
Anurādha			29:58
Ś 2			23:56
Saubhāgya			10:27
Bālava			13:15
Kaulava			23:56
Rāhu Kālam	7:56	-	9:14
Moon: Scorpio			2:19

Tuesday
5

Jyeṣṭhā			27:56
Ś 3			21:11
Śobhana			7:06
Atigaṇḍa			27:39
Taitila			10:34
Gara			21:11
Rāhu Kālam	14:27	-	15:45

Wednesday
6

Mūla			25:54
Ś 4			18:24
Sukarmā			24:12
Vanija			7:47
Viṣṭi			18:24
Bava			29:02
Rāhu Kālam	11:51	-	13:09
Moon: Sagittarius			3:56

Thursday

7

Pūrvāṣāḍhā		23:59	
Ś 5		15:42	
Dhṛti		20:50	
Bālava		15:42	
Kaulava		26:25	
Rāhu Kālam	13:08	- 14:26	

Friday

8

Uttarāṣāḍhā		22:17	
Ś 6		13:11	
Śūla		17:38	
Taitla		13:11	
Gara		24:02	
Rāhu Kālam	10:34	- 11:51	
Moon: Capricorn		5:32	Skanda Śaṣṭhī

Saturday

9

Śravaṇa		20:53	
Ś 7		10:57	
Gaṇḍa		14:41	
Vanija		10:57	
Viṣṭi		21:57	
Rāhu Kālam	9:17	- 10:34	

November 2013

S	M	T	W	T	F	S
					1	2
3	4	5	6	7	8	9
10	11	12	13	14	15	16
17	18	19	20	21	22	23
24	25	26	27	28	29	30

6	Ke 7	8	Ju 9
5			10
4			Ma 11
Ve 3	2	MeR Ra As Su Mo Sa 1	12

December 2013

S	M	T	W	T	F	S
1	2	3	4	5	6	7
8	9	10	11	12	13	14
15	16	17	18	19	20	21
22	23	24	25	26	27	28
29	30	31				

Sunday

10

Dhaniṣṭha			19:51
Ś 8			9:02
Vṛddhi			11:59
Bava			9:02
Bālava			20:13
Rāhu Kālam	15:42	-	16:58
Moon: Aquarius			8:19

Monday

Started period

11

Śatabhiṣā			19:11	
Ś 9			7:30	
Ś 10			30:32	
Dhruva			9:36	
Kaulava			7:30	
Taitila			18:53	
Gara			30:23	
Rāhu Kālam	8:02	-	9:18	Veteran's Day

Tuesday

12

Pūrva Bhādrapadā			18:56
Ś 11			29:41
Vyāghāta			7:33
Harṣaṇa			29:49
Vanija			17:59
Viṣṭi			29:41
Rāhu Kālam	14:24	-	15:40
Moon: Pisces			12:57

Wednesday

13

Uttara Bhādrapadā			19:06
Ś 12			29:25
Vajra			28:26
Bava			17:30
Bālava			29:25
Rāhu Kālam	11:52	-	13:08

Thursday
14

Revatī			19:42
Ś 13			29:36
Siddhi			27:24
Kaulava			17:27
Taitila			29:36
Rāhu Kālam	13:08	-	14:24
Moon: Aries			19:42

Friday
15

Aśvinī			20:43	
Ś 14			30:12	
Vyatīpāta			26:41	
Gara			17:51	
Vanija			30:12	
Rāhu Kālam	10:36	-	11:52	
Sun: Scorpio			22:15	Puṇya Kāla: 11:52 - 16:55

Saturday ○
16

Bharaṇī			22:09	
Pūrṇimā			Full Night	
Varīyān			26:18	
Viṣṭi			18:41	
Bava			Full Night	
Rāhu Kālam	9:21	-	10:37	Guru Nanak Jayantī • Kārttika Pūrṇimā

November 2013

S	M	T	W	T	F	S
					1	2
3	4	5	6	7	8	9
10	11	12	13	14	15	16
17	18	19	20	21	22	23
24	25	26	27	28	29	30

6	Ke 7	8	JuR 9
5			10
Mo 4			Ma 11
Ve 3	2	MeR Ra Sa As Su 1	12

December 2013

S	M	T	W	T	F	S
1	2	3	4	5	6	7
8	9	10	11	12	13	14
15	16	17	18	19	20	21
22	23	24	25	26	27	28
29	30	31				

Sunday ○
17

Kṛttikā			24:00
Pūrṇimā			7:15
Parigha			26:15
Bava			7:15
Bālava			19:56
Rāhu Kālam	15:38	-	16:53
Moon: Taurus			4:35

Monday ✱ Leaving for India!
18

Rohinī			26:14
K 1			8:43
Śiva			26:30
Kaulava			8:43
Taitila			21:37
Rāhu Kālam	8:07	-	9:22

Tuesday Should start period
19

Mṛgaśīrṣa			28:49
K 2			10:35
Siddha			27:01
Gara			10:35
Vanija			23:39
Rāhu Kālam	14:22	-	15:37
Moon: Gemini			15:29

Wednesday
20

Ārdrā			Full Night
K 3			12:48
Sādhya			27:44
Viṣṭi			12:48
Bava			26:00
Rāhu Kālam	11:53	-	13:08

Thursday
21

Ārdrā		7:39
K 4		15:15
Śubha		28:35
Bālava		15:15
Kaulava		28:32
Rāhu Kālam	13:08	- 14:22

Friday
22

Punarvasu		10:38
K 5		17:49
Śukla		29:27
Taitila		17:49
Gara		Full Night
Rāhu Kālam	10:39	- 11:54
Moon: Cancer		3:53

Saturday
23

Puṣyā		13:36
K 6		20:18
Brahma		30:12
Gara		7:04
Vanija		20:18
Rāhu Kālam	9:26	- 10:40

November 2013

S	M	T	W	T	F	S
					1	2
3	4	5	6	7	8	9
10	11	12	13	14	15	16
17	18	19	20	21	22	23
24	25	26	27	28	29	30

5	Ke 6	Mo 7	JuR 8
4			9
3			Ma 10
Ve 2	Su As 1	Me Ra Sa 12	11

December 2013

S	M	T	W	T	F	S
1	2	3	4	5	6	7
8	9	10	11	12	13	14
15	16	17	18	19	20	21
22	23	24	25	26	27	28
29	30	31				

Sunday

24

Āśleṣā			16:21
K 7			22:31
Mahendra			30:42
Viṣṭi			9:27
Bava			22:31
Rāhu Kālam	15:36	-	16:49
Moon: Leo			16:21

Monday

25

Maghā			18:42
K 8			24:15
Vaidhṛti			30:47
Bālava			11:27
Kaulava			24:15
Rāhu Kālam	8:13	-	9:27

Tuesday

26

Pūrva Phalguṇī			20:28
K 9			25:21
Viṣkambha			30:21
Taitila			12:54
Gara			25:21
Rāhu Kālam	14:22	-	15:35
Mars: Virgo			6:03

Wednesday

27

Uttara Phalguṇī			21:31	
K 10			25:42	
Prīti			29:20	
Vanija			13:37	
Viṣṭi			25:42	
Rāhu Kālam	11:55	-	13:08	Hanukah Begins

Thursday

28

Hasta		21:47
K 11		25:14
Āyuṣmān		27:41
Bava		13:34
Bālava		25:14
Rāhu Kālam	13:09 -	14:22

Thanksgiving Day

Friday

29

Citrā		21:17
K 12		23:58
Saubhāgya		25:25
Kaulava		12:42
Taitila		23:58
Rāhu Kālam	10:43 -	11:56
Moon: Libra		9:38

Saturday

30

Svāti		20:04
K 13		22:00
Śobhana		22:34
Gara		11:04
Vanija		22:00
Rāhu Kālam	9:30 -	10:43
Mercury: Scorpio		20:35

November 2013

S	M	T	W	T	F	S
					1	2
3	4	5	6	7	8	9
10	11	12	13	14	15	16
17	18	19	20	21	22	23
24	25	26	27	28	29	30

5	Ke 6	7	JuR 8
4			Mo 9
3			Ma 10
Ve 2	Su As 1	Ra Me Sa 12	11

December 2013

S	M	T	W	T	F	S
1	2	3	4	5	6	7
8	9	10	11	12	13	14
15	16	17	18	19	20	21
22	23	24	25	26	27	28
29	30	31				

Sunday
1

Viśākhā			18:14
K 14			19:25
Atigaṇḍa			19:15
Viṣṭi			8:46
Śakuni			19:25
Catuṣpada			29:56
Rāhu Kālam	15:35	-	16:47
Moon: Scorpio			12:44

Monday ●
2

Anurādha			15:55
Āmāvasyā			16:22
Sukarmā			15:32
Nāga			16:22
Kiṃsthughna			26:43
Rāhu Kālam	8:19	-	9:32

Tuesday
3

Jyeṣṭhā			13:19
Ś 1			13:01
Dhṛti			11:35
Bava			13:01
Bālava			23:17
Rāhu Kālam	14:22	-	15:35
Moon: Sagittarius			13:19

Wednesday
4

Mūla			10:35
Ś 2			9:33
Ś 3			30:08
Śūla			7:31
Gaṇḍa			27:28
Kaulava			9:33
Taitila			19:49
Gara			30:08
Rāhu Kālam	11:58	-	13:10

Thursday
5

Pūrvāṣāḍhā			7:55	
Uttarāṣāḍhā			29:28	
Ś 4			26:54	
Vṛddhi			23:34	
Vanija			16:29	
Viṣṭi			26:54	
Rāhu Kālam	13:10	-	14:23	
Moon: Capricorn			13:16	
Venus: Capricorn			0:48	Hanukah Ends

Friday
6

Śravaṇa			27:23
Ś 5			24:03
Dhruva			19:57
Bava			13:25
Bālava			24:03
Rāhu Kālam	10:46	-	11:59

Saturday
7

Dhaniṣṭhā			25:47
Ś 6			21:40
Vyāghāta			16:42
Kaulava			10:47
Taitila			21:40
Rāhu Kālam	9:35	-	10:47
Mercury: Aquarius			14:31

December 2013

S	M	T	W	T	F	S
1	2	3	4	5	6	7
8	9	10	11	12	13	14
15	16	17	18	19	20	21
22	23	24	25	26	27	28
29	30	31				

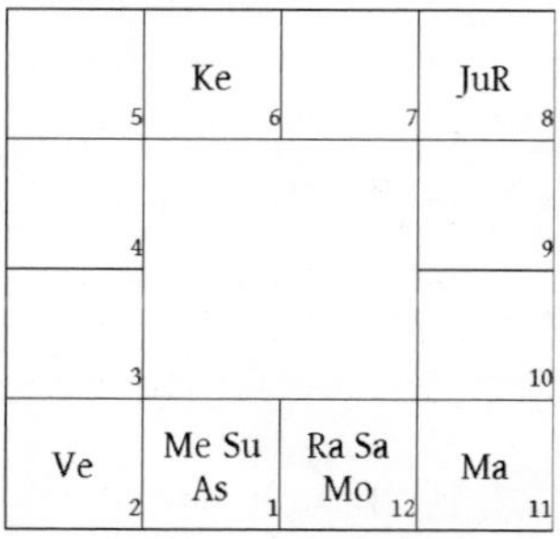

January 2014

S	M	T	W	T	F	S
			1	2	3	4
5	6	7	8	9	10	11
12	13	14	15	16	17	18
19	20	21	22	23	24	25
26	27	28	29	30	31	

Sunday

8

Śatabhiṣā		24:46
Ś 7		19:51
Harṣaṇa		13:54
Gara		8:41
Vanija		19:51
Viṣṭi		31:11
Rāhu Kālam	15:35 -	16:47

Monday

Should Start Period

9

Pūrva Bhādrapadā		24:23
Ś 8		18:41
Vajra		11:35
Bava		18:41
Bālava		30:20
Rāhu Kālam	8:25 -	9:36
Moon: Pisces		18:25

Tuesday

10

Uttara Bhādrapadā		24:37
Ś 9		18:08
Siddhi		9:47
Kaulava		18:08
Taitila		30:06
Rāhu Kālam	14:24 -	15:36

Wednesday

11

Revatī		25:25
Ś 10		18:13
Vyatīpāta		8:28
Gara		18:13
Vanija		30:28
Rāhu Kālam	12:01 -	13:13

Thursday
12

Aśvinī			26:45
Ś 11			18:51
Varīyān			7:36
Parigha			31:07
Viṣṭi			18:51
Bava			Full Night
Rāhu Kālam	13:13	-	14:24
Moon: Aries			1:25

Friday
13

Bharaṇī			28:31
Ś 12			19:58
Śiva			30:59
Bava			7:21
Bālava			19:58
Rāhu Kālam	10:50	-	12:02

Saturday
14

Kṛttikā			30:38
Ś 13			21:29
Siddha			31:07
Kaulava			8:41
Taitila			21:29
Rāhu Kālam	9:39	-	10:51
Moon: Taurus			11:01

December 2013

S	M	T	W	T	F	S
1	2	3	4	5	6	7
8	9	10	11	12	13	14
15	16	17	18	19	20	21
22	23	24	25	26	27	28
29	30	31				

5	Ke 6	7	JuR 8
Mo 4			9
Ve 3			10
2	Me As Su 1	Ra Sa 12	Ma 11

January 2014

S	M	T	W	T	F	S
			1	2	3	4
5	6	7	8	9	10	11
12	13	14	15	16	17	18
19	20	21	22	23	24	25
26	27	28	29	30	31	

Sunday 15

Rohiṇī			Full Night	
Ś 14			23:20	
Sādhya			Full Night	
Gara			10:23	
Vanija			23:20	
Rāhu Kālam	15:37	-	16:48	
Sun: Sagittarius			12:54	Puṇya Kāla: 12:54 - 18:02

Monday ○ 16

Rohiṇī			9:04
Pūrṇimā			25:28
Sādhya			7:29
Viṣṭi			12:22
Bava			25:28
Rāhu Kālam	8:29	-	9:41
Moon: Gemini			22:22

Tuesday 17

Mṛgaśīrṣa			11:43
K 1			27:48
Śubha			8:03
Bālava			14:36
Kaulava			27:48
Rāhu Kālam	14:26	-	15:38

Wednesday 18

Ārdrā			14:33
K 2			30:17
Śukla			8:45
Taitila			17:01
Gara			30:17
Rāhu Kālam	12:04	-	13:16

Thursday
19

Punarvasu		17:30
K 3		Full Night
Brahma		9:33
Vanija		19:33
Viṣṭi		Full Night
Rāhu Kālam	13:16	- 14:27
Moon: Cancer		10:45

Friday
20

Puṣyā		20:29
K 3		8:50
Mahendra		10:24
Viṣṭi		8:50
Bava		22:07
Rāhu Kālam	10:54	- 12:05
Mercury: Sagittarius		7:26

Saturday
21

Āśleṣā		23:22
K 4		11:22
Vaidhṛti		11:13
Bālava		11:22
Kaulava		24:35
Rāhu Kālam	9:43	- 10:54
Moon: Leo		23:22

Yule • Winter Solstice 9:11

December 2013

S	M	T	W	T	F	S
1	2	3	4	5	6	7
8	9	10	11	12	13	14
15	16	17	18	19	20	21
22	23	24	25	26	27	28
29	30	31				

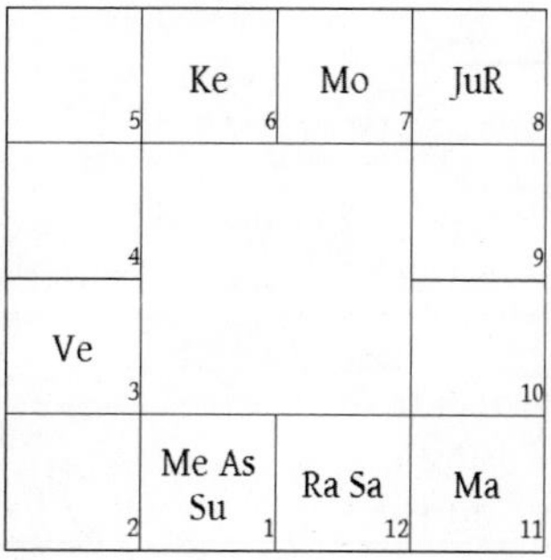

January 2014

S	M	T	W	T	F	S
			1	2	3	4
5	6	7	8	9	10	11
12	13	14	15	16	17	18
19	20	21	22	23	24	25
26	27	28	29	30	31	

Sunday

22

Maghā			26:02
K 5			13:44
Viṣkambha			11:55
Taitila			13:44
Gara			26:48
Rāhu Kālam	15:40	-	16:51

Monday

23

Pūrva Phalguṇī			28:19
K 6			15:45
Prīti			12:22
Vanija			15:45
Viṣṭi			28:35
Rāhu Kālam	8:33	-	9:44

Tuesday

24

Uttara Phalguṇī			30:01
K 7			17:16
Āyuṣman			12:28
Bava			17:16
Bālava			29:47
Rāhu Kālam	14:30	-	15:41
Moon: Virgo			10:48

Wednesday

25

Hasta			31:02	
K 8			18:07	
Saubhāgya			12:04	
Kaulava			18:07	
Taitila			30:15	
Rāhu Kālam	12:08	-	13:19	Christmas

Thursday

26

Citrā		31:14	
K 9		18:11	
Śobhana		11:06	
Gara		18:11	
Vanija		29:55	
Rāhu Kālam	13:20	- 14:31	
Moon: Libra		19:14	Kwanzaa Begins

Friday

27

Svāti		30:38
K 10		17:25
Atigaṇḍa		9:29
Sukarmā		31:13
Viṣṭi		17:25
Bava		28:43
Rāhu Kālam	10:57	- 12:09

Saturday

28

Viśākhā		29:15
K 11		15:49
Dhṛti		28:19
Bālava		15:49
Kaulava		26:44
Rāhu Kālam	9:46	- 10:58
Moon: Scorpio		23:40

December 2013

S	M	T	W	T	F	S
1	2	3	4	5	6	7
8	9	10	11	12	13	14
15	16	17	18	19	20	21
22	23	24	25	26	27	28
29	30	31				

4	Ke 5	6	JuR 7
3			8
VeR 2			Mo 9
Me As Su 1	12	Ra Sa 11	Ma 10

January 2014

S	M	T	W	T	F	S
			1	2	3	4
5	6	7	8	9	10	11
12	13	14	15	16	17	18
19	20	21	22	23	24	25
26	27	28	29	30	31	

Sunday
29

Anurādha		27:12	
K12		13:28	
Śūla		24:52	
Taitila		13:28	
Gara		24:03	
Rāhu Kālam	15:44	- 16:56	

Monday
30

Jyeṣṭhā		24:36	
K 13		10:29	
K 14		31:00	
Gaṇḍa		20:57	
Vanija		10:29	
Viṣṭi		20:47	
Śakuni		31:00	
Rāhu Kālam	8:35	- 9:47	

Tuesday ●
31

Mūla		21:38	
Āmāvasyā		27:14	
Vṛddhi		16:43	
Catuṣpada		17:09	
Nāga		27:14	
Rāhu Kālam	14:34	- 15:46	
Moon: Sagittarius		0:36	New Year's Eve

Wednesday
1

Pūrvāṣāḍhā		18:31	
Ś 1		23:21	
Dhruva		12:20	
Kiṃsthughna		13:18	
Bava		23:20	
Rāhu Kālam	12:12	- 13:24	
Moon: Capricorn		23:43	New Year's Day • Kwanzaa Ends

Thursday
2

Uttarāṣāḍhā			15:26
Ś 2			19:33
Vyāghāta			7:54
Harṣaṇa			27:37
Bālava			9:25
Kaulava			19:32
Taitila			29:42
Rāhu Kālam	13:24	-	14:36

Friday
3

Śravaṇa			12:34
Ś 3			16:02
Vajra			23:36
Gara			16:01
Vanija			26:24
Rāhu Kālam	11:01	-	12:13
Moon: Aquarius			23:18

Saturday
4

Dhaniṣṭha			10:09
Ś 4			12:57
Siddhi			20:02
Viṣṭi			12:56
Bava			23:38
Rāhu Kālam	9:49	-	11:01
Moon: Scorpio			23:40

December 2013

S	M	T	W	T	F	S
1	2	3	4	5	6	7
8	9	10	11	12	13	14
15	16	17	18	19	20	21
22	23	24	25	26	27	28
29	30	31				

4	Ke 5	6	JuR 7
3			8
VeR 2			9
As Su Me 1	Mo 12	Ra Sa 11	Ma 10

January 2014

S	M	T	W	T	F	S
			1	2	3	4
5	6	7	8	9	10	11
12	13	14	15	16	17	18
19	20	21	22	23	24	25
26	27	28	29	30	31	

Sunday
5

Śatabhiṣā			8:19
Ś 5			10:30
Vyatīpāta			16:58
Bālava			10:29
Kaulava			21:39
Rāhu Kālam	15:50	-	17:03

Monday
6

Pūrva Bhādrapadā			7:12
Ś 6			8:46
Varīyān			14:31
Taitila			8:45
Gara			20:11
Śakuni			31:00
Rāhu Kālam	8:37	-	9:49
Moon: Pisces			1:23
Venus: Sagittarius			10:02

Tuesday
7

Uttara Bhādrapadā			6:50
Ś 7			7:50
Parigha			12:43
Vanija			7:49
Viṣṭi			19:39
Rāhu Kālam	14:40	-	15:52
Moon: Sagittarius			0:36
Mercury: Capricorn			23:48

Wednesday
8

Revatī			7:15
Ś 8			7:42
Śiva			11:31
Bava			7:41
Bālava			19:54
Rāhu Kālam	12:15	-	13:28
Moon: Aries			7:15

Thursday
9

Aśvinī			8:26
Ś 9			8:18
Siddha			10:52
Kaulva			8:18
Taitila			20:51
Rāhu Kālam	13:28	-	14:41

Friday
10

Bharaṇī			10:12
Ś 10			9:35
Sādhya			10:44
Gara			9:34
Vanija			22:24
Rāhu Kālam	11:03	-	12:16
Moon: Taurus			16:44

Saturday
11

Kṛttikā			12:27
Ś 11			11:21
Śubha			10:58
Viṣṭi			11:20
Bava			24:22
Rāhu Kālam	9:50	-	11:03

January 2014

S	M	T	W	T	F	S
			1	2	3	4
5	6	7	8	9	10	11
12	13	14	15	16	17	18
19	20	21	22	23	24	25
26	27	28	29	30	31	

4	Ke 5	6	JuR 7
Mo 3			8
VeR 2			9
As Su Me 1	12	Ra Sa 11	Ma 10

February 2014

S	M	T	W	T	F	S
			1	2	1	2
3	4	5	6	7	8	9
10	11	12	13	14	15	16
17	18	19	20	21	22	23
24	25	26	27	28		

Daily Sunrise and Sunset Timings for San Ramon, California

	1	2	3	4	5	6	7	8	9	10	11	12	13	14	15
Jan	7:24-16:58	7:24-16:59	7:24-17:00	7:25-17:01	7:25-17:02	7:25-17:03	7:24-17:04	7:24-17:05	7:24-17:06	7:24-17:07	7:24-17:08	7:24-17:09	7:24-17:10	7:23-17:11	7:23-17:12
Feb	7:12-17:30	7:11-17:31	7:11-17:33	7:10-17:34	7:09-17:35	7:08-17:36	7:07-17:37	7:06-17:38	7:05-17:39	7:04-17:40	7:02-17:41	7:01-17:42	7:00-17:44	6:59-17:45	6:58-17:46
Mar	6:40-18:00	6:38-18:01	6:37-18:02	6:35-18:03	6:34-18:04	6:32-18:05	6:31-18:06	6:30-16:26	6:28-18:08	7:27-19:09	7:25-19:10	7:24-19:11	7:22-19:12	7:21-19:13	7:19-19:14
Apr	6:53-19:30	6:52-19:30	6:50-19:31	6:49-19:32	6:47-19:33	6:46-19:34	6:44-19:35	6:43-19:36	6:42-19:37	6:40-19:38	6:39-19:39	6:37-19:40	6:36-19:40	6:34-19:41	6:33-19:42
May	6:12-19:57	6:11-19:58	6:10-19:59	6:09-20:00	6:08-20:01	6:07-20:02	6:06-20:02	6:05-20:03	6:04-20:04	6:03-20:05	6:02-20:06	6:01-20:07	6:00-20:08	5:59-20:09	5:59-20:10
Jun	5:48-20:23	5:48-20:23	5:48-20:24	5:47-20:25	5:47-20:25	5:47-20:26	5:47-20:27	5:46-20:27	5:46-20:28	5:46-20:28	5:46-20:29	5:46-20:29	5:46-20:29	5:46-20:30	5:46-20:30
Jul	5:51-20:32	5:51-20:32	5:52-20:32	5:52-20:31	5:53-20:31	5:53-20:31	5:54-20:31	5:54-20:30	5:55-20:30	5:56-20:30	5:56-20:29	5:57-20:29	5:58-20:29	5:58-20:28	5:59-20:28
Aug	6:12-20:14	6:13-20:13	6:14-20:12	6:15-20:11	6:16-20:10	6:17-20:09	6:18-20:08	6:18-20:07	6:19-20:06	6:20-20:05	6:21-20:04	6:22-20:02	6:23-20:01	6:24-20:00	6:24-19:59
Sep	6:39-19:35	6:40-19:33	6:41-19:32	6:41-19:30	6:42-19:29	6:43-19:27	6:44-19:26	6:45-19:24	6:46-19:23	6:47-19:21	6:47-19:20	6:48-19:18	6:49-19:17	6:50-19:15	6:51-19:14
Oct	7:04-18:49	7:05-18:47	7:06-18:46	7:07-18:44	7:08-18:43	7:09-18:41	7:10-18:40	7:11-18:38	7:12-18:37	7:13-18:35	7:14-18:34	7:14-18:33	7:15-18:31	7:16-18:30	7:17-18:28
Nov	7:34-18:07	7:35-18:06	6:36-17:05	6:38-17:04	6:39-17:03	6:40-17:02	6:41-17:01	6:42-17:00	6:43-16:59	6:44-16:59	6:45-16:58	6:46-16:57	6:47-16:56	6:48-16:55	6:49-16:55
Dec	7:06-16:47	7:07-16:47	7:08-16:47	7:08-16:47	7:09-16:47	7:10-16:47	7:11-16:47	7:12-16:47	7:13-16:47	7:14-16:47	7:14-16:47	7:15-16:48	7:16-16:48	7:16-16:48	7:17-16:48

Daily Sunrise and Sunset Timings for San Ramon, California

	16	17	18	19	20	21	22	23	24	25	26	27	28	29	30	31
Jan	7:22- 17:13	7:22- 17:14	7:22- 17:15	7:21- 17:16	7:21- 17:17	7:20- 17:18	7:20- 17:19	7:19- 17:20	7:18- 17:21	7:18- 17:22	7:17- 17:24	7:16- 17:25	7:16- 17:26	7:15- 17:27	7:14- 17:28	7:13- 17:29
Feb	6:57- 17:47	6:56- 17:48	6:54- 17:49	6:53- 17:50	6:52- 17:51	6:50- 17:52	6:49- 17:53	6:48- 17:54	6:46- 17:55	6:45- 17:56	6:44- 17:57	6:42- 17:58	6:41- 17:59			
Mar	7:18- 19:15	7:16- 19:16	7:15- 19:17	7:13- 19:18	7:12- 19:19	7:10- 19:19	7:09- 19:20	7:07- 19:21	7:05- 19:22	7:04- 19:23	7:02- 19:24	7:01- 19:25	6:59- 19:26	6:58- 19:27	6:56- 19:28	6:54- 19:29
Apr	6:32- 19:43	6:30- 19:44	6:29- 19:45	6:28- 19:46	6:26- 19:47	6:25- 19:48	6:24- 19:49	6:22- 19:50	6:21- 19:51	6:20- 19:51	6:18- 19:52	6:17- 19:53	6:16- 19:54	6:15- 19:55	6:14- 19:56	
May	5:58- 20:10	5:57- 20:11	5:56- 20:12	5:55- 20:13	5:55- 20:14	5:54- 20:15	5:53- 20:15	5:53- 20:16	5:52- 20:17	5:52- 20:18	5:51- 20:18	5:50- 20:19	5:50- 20:20	5:50- 20:21	5:49- 20:21	5:49- 20:22
Jun	5:46- 20:30	5:46- 20:31	5:47- 20:31	5:47- 20:31	5:47- 20:31	5:47- 20:31	5:47- 20:32	5:48- 20:32	5:48- 20:32	5:48- 20:32	5:49- 20:32	5:49- 20:32	5:49- 20:32	5:50- 20:32	5:50- 20:32	
Jul	6:00- 20:27	6:00- 20:26	6:01- 20:26	6:02- 20:25	6:03- 20:24	6:03- 20:24	6:04- 20:23	6:05- 20:22	6:06- 20:22	6:07- 20:21	6:07- 20:20	6:08- 20:19	6:09- 20:18	6:10- 20:17	6:11- 20:16	6:12- 20:15
Aug	6:25- 19:57	6:26- 19:56	6:27- 19:55	6:28- 19:53	6:29- 19:52	6:30- 19:51	6:30- 19:49	6:31- 19:48	6:32- 19:47	6:33- 19:45	6:34- 19:44	6:35- 19:42	6:36- 19:41	6:36- 19:39	6:37- 19:37	6:38- 19:36
Sep	6:52- 19:12	6:52- 19:10	6:53- 19:09	6:54- 19:07	6:55- 19:06	6:56- 19:04	6:57- 19:03	6:57- 19:01	6:58- 19:00	6:59- 18:58	7:00- 18:56	7:01- 18:55	7:02- 18:53	7:03- 15:52	7:04- 18:50	
Oct	7:18- 18:27	7:19- 18:26	7:20- 18:24	7:21- 18:23	7:22- 18:22	7:23- 18:20	7:24- 18:19	7:25- 18:18	7:26- 18:16	7:27- 18:15	7:28- 18:14	7:29- 18:13	7:30- 18:12	7:31- 18:11	7:32- 18:09	7:33- 18:08
Nov	6:50- 16:54	6:51- 16:53	6:52- 16:53	6:54- 16:52	6:55- 16:51	6:56- 16:51	6:57- 16:50	6:58- 16:50	6:59- 16:49	7:00- 16:49	7:01- 16:49	7:02- 16:48	7:03- 16:48	7:04- 16:48	7:05- 16:48	
Dec	7:18- 16:49	7:18- 16:49	7:19- 16:50	7:20- 16:50	7:20- 16:50	7:21- 16:51	7:21- 16:51	7:22- 16:52	7:22- 16:53	7:22- 16:53	7:23- 16:54	7:23- 16:54	7:23- 16:55	7:24- 16:56	7:24- 1657	7:24- 16:57

108 Names of Dakṣiṇāmūrti

Dakṣiṇāmūrti Aṣṭottaraśata Nāmavāliḥ

1. Oṁ Mahādevāya Namaḥ
   Salutations to God supreme.
2. Oṁ Adi guru sthitāya Namaḥ
   Salutations to the he who is the foremost amongst spiritual teachers.
3. Oṁ Hrīṁ kāra rūpāya Namaḥ
   Salutations to he whose form is the mantra Hrīṁ.
4. Oṁ Maunena phalo ttama pradāya Namaḥ
   Salutations to he who gives the ultimate fruit (liberation) through the medium of silence.
5. Oṁ Jñāna jñatṛ jñeyāya Namaḥ
   Salutaions to he who is the knower, that which is to be known as well as the knowledge itself.
6. Oṁ Strī puruṣa manikarnikāya Namaḥ
   Salutations to he who has a male and female earring in his left and right ear (Ārdhanārīśvara).
7. Oṁ Chaṇḍas puraṇe tihāsa paribbhujāya Namaḥ
   Salutations to he who the protector all of the sacred scriptures.
8. Oṁ Turīyātītāya Namaḥ
   Salutations to he who is above the states of waking, sleep, dreamless sleep and the fourth state which transcends all others.
9. Oṁ Dvaita advaita saṁśayāya Namaḥ
   Salutations to he who destroys duality, non-duality and every thing in between.
10. Oṁ Nandīśādimadeśikāya Namaḥ
    Salutations to the Lord of the foremost of devotees, Nandīśvara

11. Oṁ Mohānalasudhā sārāya Namaḥ
Salutations to he who pours nectar to extinguish the fire of delusion.
12. Oṁ Mohāmbuja sudhākarāya Namaḥ
Salutations to he who acts like the full Moon which closes the lotus of delusion.
13. Oṁ Mohāndhakāra taraṇaye Namaḥ
Salutations to he who is the Sun, illuminating the darkness of delusion.
14. Oṁ Mohot-palana-bhomaṇaye Namaḥ
Salutations to he who is the Sun which causes the water-lily of ignorance to mature.
15. Oṁ Bhakta jñānābdhi śītāṁśave Namaḥ
Salutations to he who is the ocean of Knowledge for his devotees.
16. Oṁ Bhakta keki ghanāghanāya Namaḥ
Salutations to the one who is fire to the straw bed of ignorance of the devotees.
17. Oṁ Bhaktāmbhoja sahasraṁśave Namaḥ
Salutations to the one who is the Sun that opens the lotus heart of his devotees.
18. Oṁ Bhakta keki ṭṭanāṭṭanāya Namaḥ
Salutations to the one who causes joy to spring up within his devotees like peacocks dancing in the rain.
19. Oṁ Bhakta kairava rākendave Namaḥ
Salutations to he who causes his devotees hearts to blossom like a white lily flower.
20. Oṁ Bhakta kokadi vākarāya Namaḥ
Salutations to he who dispels the longing of the devotees like the rising Sun does for the Cakravāka bird.*

*The poetic Cakravāka bird deeply longs and yearns for the sunrise and can't find solace until it can bathe in it's golden rays.

21. Oṁ Gajanana adi sampūjyāya Namaḥ
    Salutations to he who is worshipped by Gaṇeśa as well as other chief devotees.
22. Oṁ Gajacarm ojjvala-akṛtaye Namaḥ
    Salutations to he who wears the elephant skin of slain desire.
23. Oṁ Gaṅgā dhavala divyāṅgāya Namaḥ
    Salutations to he who is carries the purifying Ganges river on his head.
24. Oṁ Gaṅgā paṅki lasajjaṭāya Namaḥ
    Salutations to he with holy clay from the Ganges banks caked in his matted hair.
25. Oṁ Gagana-ambara saṁvītāya Namaḥ
    Salutations to he who uses space itself as his wearing cloth.
26. Oṁ Gaganā mukta mūrdhajāya Namaḥ
    Salutations to he who wears his matted locks like clouds in the sky.
27. Oṁ Vadanābja jitābja śriye Namaḥ
    Salutations to he whose beauty surpasses a fully blossomed lotus flower.
28. Oṁ Vadanendu sphurad diśāya Namaḥ
    Salutations to he whose form brightens the four quarters of the earth.
29. Oṁ Varadā naika nipuṇāya Namaḥ
    Salutations to the one who is the supreme authority for granting boons.
30. Oṁ Varavīṇ ojjvalat karāya Namaḥ
    Salutations to he who holds an excellent *vīna*, a stringed instrument, in his hands.
31. Oṁ Vanavāsa samullāsāya Namaḥ
    Salutations to he who delights in dwelling in the forest, away from sense pleasures.

32. Oṁ Vana vīraika lolupāya Namaḥ

Salutations to he who deeply longs for the company of other forest dwellers, those who also isolate themselves from the fruit of sense pleasures.

33. Oṁ Tejaḥ phullaṇktana-akārāya Namaḥ

Salutations to he whose dazzling form is surrounded by the light of the Self.

34. Oṁ Tejasāmapi bhāsakāya Namaḥ

Salutations to the one who illumines the heavenly bodies of Sun and Moon.

35. Oṁ Vineyānāṁ tejaḥ pradāya Namaḥ

Salutations to he who gives this brilliance to the humble.

36. Oṁ Tejomaya nijāśramāya Namaḥ

Salutations to he whose dwelling place is completely awash with lustre.

37. Oṁ Damita-anaṅga saṁgrāmāya Namaḥ

Salutations to he who has completely conquered desire.

38. Oṁ Darahā sajita-aṅganāya Namaḥ

Salutations to he who won over Umā with a gentle smile.

39. Oṁ Dayārasa sudhā sindhave Namaḥ

Salutations to he who is a brimming ocean of pure compassion.

40. Oṁ Daridra dhana śevadhaye Namaḥ

Salutations to the one who serves the poor.

41. Oṁ Kṣīrendu sphaṭikā kārāya Namaḥ

Salutations to him whose form is pure like that of milk, the Moon or a crystal.

42. Oṁ Kṣīrendu mukuṭ ojjvalāya Namaḥ

Salutations to him whose crown is resplendent like the full milky white Moon.

43. Oṁ Kṣīropahā rarasikāya Namaḥ

Salutations to the one who relishes milk offered by the devotee.

44. Oṁ Kṣipraiśvarya phala pradāya Namaḥ
Salutations to he who grants the opulence of Self Knowledge readily.

45. Oṁ Nānā bharaṇa mugdha aṅgāya Namaḥ
Salutations to the one who is bedecked with ornaments.

46. Oṁ Nārīsam mohanā kṛtaye Namaḥ
Salutation to he whose beautiful form as the very Self of all, enchants creation.

47. Oṁ Nāda brahma rasāsvādine Namaḥ
Salutations to he who delights in divine music.

48. Oṁ Nāga bhūṣaṇa bhūṣitāya Namaḥ
Salutations to the one who is adorned with serpents, who has conquered worldly desire.

49. Oṁ Mūrti nindita kandarpāya Namaḥ
Salutations to he whose beauty surpasses even that of Manmatha, the God of love.

50. Oṁ Mūrtā mūrta jagad vapuṣe Namaḥ
Salutations to he whose body is the very Universe that is made of the five elements.

51. Oṁ Mūlājñāna tamobhānave Namaḥ
Salutations to he who destroys the inert root of ignorance in his devotees

52. Oṁ Mūrtimat kalpa pādāya Namaḥ
Salutations to he who is the wish-fulfilling tree of desire for his devotees.

53. Oṁ Taruṇ āditya saṅkāśāya Namaḥ
Salutations to he who is like the morning Sun.

54. Oṁ Tantrī vādana tat parāya Namaḥ
Salutations to the one who delights in the playing of the vīṇā.

55. Oṁ Taru mūlaika nilayāya Namaḥ
Salutations to he who is seated under the banyan tree, apart from māyā.

56. Oṁ Tapta jāmbūnada prabhāya Namaḥ

Salutations to he whose body is radiant and glowing like the celestial river Jāmbūnaḍī.

57. Oṁ Tatva pusto llasat pāṇaye Namaḥ

Salutations to he who holds the holy Veda in his hand.

58. Oṁ Tapan oḍupa locanāya Namaḥ

Salutations to he whose eyes verily are the Sun and Moon.

59. Oṁ Yama sannu tasat kīrtaye Namaḥ

Salutations to he whose divinity is sung by even Yama Mahārāja.

60. Oṁ Yama saṁyama saṅyutāya Namaḥ

Salutations to he who is endowed with the six yamas as well as the three saṁyamas.*

61. Oṁ Yatirūpa dharāya Namaḥ

Salutations to he who is in the form of a sincere spiritual ascetic.

62. Oṁ Yatīndro pāsya vigrahāya Namaḥ

Salutations to he whose form is meditated upon by devout spiritual aspirants.

63. Oṁ Mandāra hāra rucirāya Namaḥ

Salutations to the one who looks beautiful bedecked with the crimson starburst flower.

64. Oṁ Madanā huta sundarāya Namaḥ

Salutation to he whose beauty surpasses even 1,000 Cupids.

65. Oṁ Mandasmita lasad vaktrāya Namaḥ

Salutations to he whose gentle smile moves coyly about his face.

66. Oṁ Madhurā dhara pallavāya Namaḥ

Salutations to the one with a sweet, flower bud-like lower lip.

67. Oṁ Mañjīra mañju pādābjāya Namaḥ

Salutations to the one with lovely anklets adorning his lotus feet.

*The six Yamas are Ahimsā - non violence, Satya - truthfulness, Asteya - not stealing, Brahmācārya - a chaste life, Aparigraha - absence of greed, Śauca - cleanliness. The three Saṃyamas are Dhāraṇā - concentration, Dhyāna - contemplation, Samādhi - absorption.

68. Oṁ Maṇipaṭṭo lasatkaṭaye Namaḥ
Salutations to the one whose waist belt is bedazzled with gems.

69. Oṁ Hasta-ahlurita cinmudrāya Namaḥ
Salutations to he who teaches supreme Reality with the Cin Mudra.

70. Oṁ Haṭhayoga parottamāya Namaḥ
Salutations to the Supreme Lord who practices Hatha Yoga.

71. Oṁ Haṁsa jāpyakṣa mālāḍhyāya Namaḥ
Salutations to he who chants the *So-Haṁ* mantra on his rosary.

72. Oṁ Haṁsendrā rādhya pādukāya Namaḥ
Salutations to he whose sandals are worshipped by the Knowers of the Self.

73. Oṁ Meru śṛṅga taṭollāsāya Namaḥ
Salutations to the one who resides in the celestial peaks of Mount Meru.

74. Oṁ Meṭṭaśyāma manoharāya Namaḥ
Salutations to he who captivates even the heart of Viṣṇu Bhagavān.

75. Oṁ Meṭṭāṅkurā lavālā gryāya Namaḥ
Salutations to he who is the very source of the Intellect.

76. Oṁ Medhā pakva phala drumāya Namaḥ
Salutations to the one who yields the ripe fruit of unmatchable Intellect.

77. Oṁ Dhārmika-antar guhā vāsāya Namaḥ
Salutations to he whose abode is in the heart of the righteous.

78. Oṁ Dharma mārga pravartakāya Namaḥ
Salutations to he who promotes the path of righteousness.

79. Oṁ Dhāma traya nijārāmāya Namaḥ
Salutations to he with his abode as Sat-Cit-Ānanda.

80. Oṁ Dharmottama mano rathāya Namaḥ
Salutation to the one worshipped by the sages committed to Self Knowledge.

81. Oṁ Prabodho drāra dīpaśriye Namaḥ
Salutations to that foremost teacher who pours our Knowledge like a lamp emits light.
82. Oṁ Prakaśita jagat trayāya Namaḥ
Salutations to that one who illumines both the underworld and earth as well as heaven to be illumined.
83. Oṁ Prajñā candraśilā candrāya Namaḥ
Salutations to the one who is both the Moon and moon-stone of pure Knowledge.
84. Oṁ Prajñā maṇi varākarāya Namaḥ
Salutations to he who is the precious jewel of Intellect and Knowledge.
85. Oṁ Jñāna-anantara thnāsātmane Namaḥ
Salutations to he who shines as Consciousness that exist between two thoughts.
86. Oṁ Jñātṛ jñānādi vidūragāya Namaḥ
Salutations to the one who is the Knower, that which is to be known as well as the act of knowing.
87. Oṁ Jñānajña-advaita divyāṅgāya Namaḥ
Salutations to the one who shines with the brilliance of Knowledge.
88. Oṁ Jñātṛ jñānādi kulāgatāya Namaḥ
Salutations to the one whose very nature pervades the knower, knowledge and that which is to be known.
89. Oṁ Prapanna pārijātāgryāya Namaḥ
Salutations to the one who is foremost in fulfilling the desires of those who take refuge in him.
90. Oṁ Prāṇata-artya-abdhi vāḍavāya Namaḥ
Salutations to he who is like a life-raft in the ocean of suffering.
91. Oṁ Bhūtānāṁ pramāṇa bhūtāya Namaḥ
Salutations to the one who is the very essence of the substance of existence.

92. Oṁ Prapañca hita kārakāya Namaḥ

Salutations to he who is the supporter of the world.

93. Oṁ Yat tat-tvam-asi saṁvedhyāya Namaḥ

Salutations to he who completely reveals the Self through the divine saying, "Thou art *That*".

94. Oṁ Yakṣa geyātma vaibhavāya Namaḥ

Salutations to he whose praises were beautifully sung by the god of wealth, Kubera.

95. Oṁ Yajñādi devatā mūrtye Namaḥ

Salutations to he who partakes first at ritual sacrifices.

96. Oṁ Yajamāna vapurdharāya Namaḥ

Salutations to he who manifests himself as the officiator of Vedic ceremonies.

97. Oṁ Chatrādhipati viśveśāya Namaḥ

Salutations to he who is Lord of all the rulers of the earth.

98. Oṁ Chatra cāmara sevitāya Namaḥ

Salutations to he who is served with fans and an umbrella.

99. Oṁ Chandaś śāstrādi nipuṇāya Namaḥ

Salutations to him who is the very knowledge of the Veda and it's axillary limbs.

100. Oṁ Chalajātyādi dūragāya Namaḥ

Salutations to he who keeps his distance from fraud and false logicians.

101. Oṁ Svābhāvika sukhaika-atmane Namaḥ

Salutations to he whose inner nature is the peace that arises from the Self alone.

102. Oṁ Svānu bhūti raso dadhaye Namaḥ

Salutations to the one who is very nature is an ocean of joy.

103. Oṁ Svārājya sampadadhya kṣāya Namaḥ

Salutations to he who presides over an inner nature of freedom.

104. Oṁ Svātmā rāma mahā mataye Namaḥ

Salutations to he who naturally abides in the Self as complete knowledge.

105. Oṁ Hāṭakā bhajaṭā jūṭāya Namaḥ
Salutations to he whose matted locks gleam with brilliance like pure gold.

106. Oṁ Hāsodastāri maṇḍalāya Namaḥ
Salutations to he who completely disarms enemies with his smile.

107. Oṁ Hālāhal ojjavala galāya Namaḥ
Salutations to he who is a master over his sense organs.

108. Oṁ Hārda granthi vimocakāya Namaḥ
Salutations to he who unbinds the knot of the heart of his devotees.

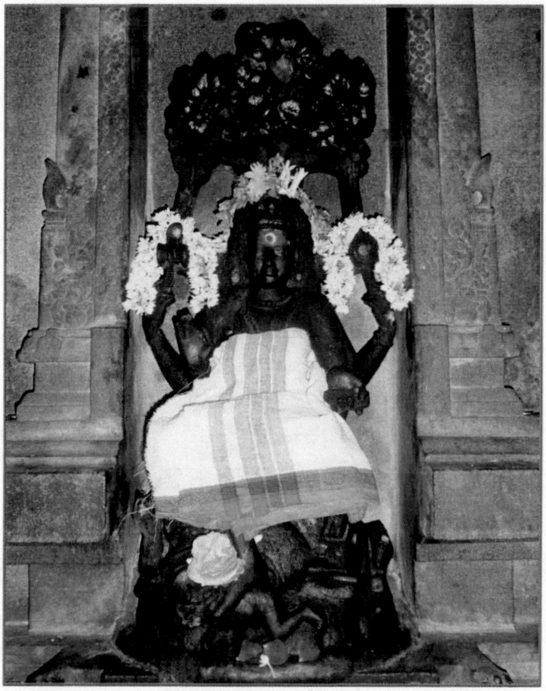

Dakṣiṇāmūrti statue from the temple in Ramana Mahārṣi's Aśrama

Dakṣiṇāmūrti Stotram

Oṁ Hrīṁ dakṣiṇāmūrtaye tubhyaṁ vaṭa mūla nivāsine |
Dhyānaika niratāṅgāya namo rudrāya śambhave Hrīṁ Oṁ || मूल ||

Vaṭa viṭapi samīpe bhūmibhāge niṣaṇṇaṁ |
Sakala muni janānāṁ jñāna dātā ramārāt || पूर्व 1 ||

Tribhuvana gurumīśaṁ dakṣiṇāmūrti devaṁ |
Janana maraṇa duḥkha ccheda dakṣaṁ namāmi || पूर्व 2 ||

Citraṁ vaṭataror mūle vṛddhāḥ śiṣyā gururyuvā |
Gurostu maunaṁ vyākhyānaṁ śiṣyāstu chinnasaṁśayāḥ || पूर्व 3 ||

Nidhaye sarva vidyānāṁ bhiṣaje bhāva rogiṇām |
Gurave sarva lokānāṁ dakṣiṇāmūrtaye namaḥ || पूर्व 4 ||

Oṁ namaḥ praṇavārthāya śuddha jñānaika mūrtaye |
Nirmalāya praśāntāya dakṣiṇāmūrtaye namaḥ || पूर्व 5 ||

Mauna vyākhyā parkaṭita parabrahma tattvaṁ yuvānaṁ
Varṣiṣtha antevasa dṛṣigaṇair āvṛtaṁ brahma niṣṭhaiḥ |
Ācāryendraṁ karakalita cinmudram ānanda rūpaṁ
Svātmārāmaṁ mudita vadanaṁ dakṣiṇāmūrtimīḍe || 1 ||

Viśvaṃ darpaṇadṛśyamānanagarītulyaṃ nijāntargataṃ
Paśyannātmani māyayā bahirivodbhūtaṃ yathā nidrayā |
Yaḥ sākṣāt kurute prabodha samaye svātmānam evā dvayaṃ
Tasmai śrīgurumūrtaye nama idaṃ śrīdakṣiṇāmūrtaye || 2 ||

Bījasya antariva aṅkuro jagadidaṃ prāṅnirvikalpaṁ punaḥ
Māyākalpitadeśakālakalanāvaicitryacitrīkṛtam |
Māyāvīva vijṛmbhayatyapi mahāyogīva yaḥ svecchayā
tasmai śrīgurumūrtaye nama idaṃ śrīdakṣiṇāmūrtaye || 3 ||

Yasyaiva sphuraṇaṃ sadātmakam asat kalpārthagaṃ bhāsate
Sākṣāt tattvamas īti vedavacasā yo bodhayat yāśritān |
Yat sākṣāt karaṇād bhavenna punara avṛttir bhavām bhonidhau
Tasmai śrīgurumūrtaye nama idaṃ śrīdakṣiṇāmūrtaye || 4 ||

Nānā chidra ghaṭo dara sthita mahā dīpa prabhā bhāsvaraṁ
Jñānaṃ yasya tu cakṣurādi karaṇad vārā bahiḥ spandate |
Jānāmīti tameva bhāntam anubhātye tat samaṣtaṃ jagat
Tasmai śrīgurumūrtaye nama idaṃ śrīdakṣiṇāmūrtaye || 5 ||

Dehaṃ prāṇamap īndriyāṇyapi calāṃ buddhiṃ ca śūnyaṃ viduḥ
Śrī bāla andhajaḍo pamāstv aham iti bhrāntā bhṛśaṃ vādinaḥ |
Māyā śaktivilāsa kalpita mahāvyāmoha saṃhāriṇe
Tasmai śrīgurumūrtaye nama idaṃ śrīdakṣiṇāmūrtaye || 6 ||

Rāhugrasta divākar endusadṛśo māyā samācchādanāt
Sanmātraḥ karaṇo pasaṃharaṇato yo'bhūt suṣuptaḥ pumān |
Prāgasvāpsam iti prabodha samaye yaḥ pratya bhijñāyate
Tasmai śrīgurumūrtaye nama idaṃ śrīdakṣiṇāmūrtaye || 7 ||

Bālyādi ṣvapi jāgradādiṣu tathā sarvā svavasthā svapi
Vyāvṛttā svanuvartamāna mahamityantaḥ sphurantaṁ sadā |
Svātmānaṃ prakaṭīkaroti bhajatāṃ yo mudrayā bhadrayā
Tasmai śrīgurūmūrtaye nama idaṃ śrīdakṣaṇoomūrtaye || 8 ||

Viśvaṃ paśyati kārya kāraṇatayā svasvāmisambandhataḥ
Śiṣyācārya tayā tathaiva pitṛ putra adyātmanā bhedataḥ |
Svapne jāgrati vā ya eṣa puruṣo māyā paribhrāmitaḥ
Tasmai śrigurumūrtaye nama idaṃ śrīdakṣiṇāmūrtaye || 9 ||

Bhūram bhāṁsya nalo-nilo –mbaramahar
nātho himāṃśuḥ pumān
Ityābhāti caracara atmakamidaṃ yasyaiva mūrtyaṣṭakam |
Nānyatkiñcana vidyate vimṛśatāṃ yasmāt parasmādvibhoḥ
Tasmai śrīgurumūrtaye nama idaṃ śrīdakṣiṇāmūrtaye || 10 ||

Sarva atmatvam iti sphuṭī kṛtam idaṃ yasmād amuṣmin stave
Tenāsya śravaṇāt tadartha mananād dhyānācca saṅkīrtanāt |
Sarva atmatvamahā vibhūti sahitaṃ syād īśvaratvaṃ svataḥ
Siddhyet tat punar aṣṭadhā pariṇataṃ caiśvaryam avyāhatam || 11 ||

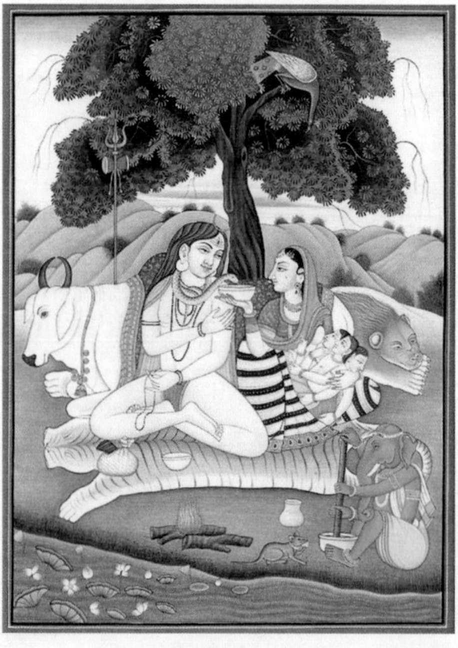

Quick and Easy Pronunciation Guide for Transliterated Sanskrit

For the words appearing in Kālāmṛta

A as in apparent

Ā as in father

I as in ink

Ī as in email

U as in pull

Ū as in pool

Ṛ as in rhythm

E as in date

Ai as in piety

O as in ocean

Au as in outside

C as in chaste

Ṅ as in pang

Ñ as in b-ungee cord

Ṇ as in bandana

Ṁ as in bum, dam or dim

Ṣ and **Ś** though the mechanics of pronunciation are different, to the western ear they have similar sounds as in Shampoo.

Ḍ, Ṣ and **Ṭ** are pronounced with the tongue touching the roof of the mouth

Ḍ as in drum

Ṭ as in true

Glossary

Abhijit Muhūrta: a generally auspicious time of day, when the Sun is directly overhead. A 48 minute duration of time

Air hand: have square palms, long fingers, soft skin with thin, deep lines that look wispy and elegant. The typical fingerprint pattern for an air hand is the loop.

Ākrama Rekhā: attaining, approaching, obtaining and overcoming; the "Simian line".

Akṣaya Tṛtīya: is on May 12. One of the four most auspicious days of the year for Muhūrta; occurs on the third Tithi of Śukla Pakṣa when the Sun is in Aries and the Moon is in Taurus.

Āmāvasyā: the thirtieth Tithi. The darkest Tithi ends with the exact New Moon.

Amma's Birthday: is celebrated on September 27th.

Annular eclipse: a solar eclipse which occurs when a portion of the Sun's surface is visible as a ring surrounding the dark Moon.

Anurādha: the seventeenth Nakṣatra.

Arch fingerprints: look just like an arch, like a low wave in the lines that make up the fingerprints. They are the simplest (and rarest) fingerprint pattern.

Ārdrā: the sixth Nakṣatra.

Aruṇācala: a mythical as well as literal mountain in the South Indian state of Tamiḷ Nadu, about 200 km South-West of Chennai.

Āśleṣā: the ninth Nakṣatra.

Aṣṭamī: the eighth Tithi.

Aśvinī: the first Nakṣatra.

Ātmā: the Self of All.

Ātmā jñāna: knowledge of the Self of All.

Ayanāmśa: lit. "Moving portion"; the difference between the tropical and sidereal zodiacs.

Bharaṇī: the second Nakṣatra.

Brahma Muhūrta: the 48 minute period just before sunrise.

Bṛhat Saṃhitā: an ancient text by the astrologer Vārāhamihīra.

Candra Balā: lit. "Strength of the Moon"; refers to the relationship be tween one's natal Moon position and the position of the Moon in the heavens on a given day.

Caturthī: the fourth Tithi.

Caturdaśī: the fourteenth Tithi.

Cin Mudra: a hand gesture made by Dakṣiṇāmūrti where the hand is held upright – palm out – and the thumb holds down the bent first finger while the middle, ring and baby finger remain erect.

Citrā: the fourteenth Nakṣatra.

Dakṣiṇāmūrti: An incarnation of Lord Śiva in the form of the silent, Supreme Teacher.

Dakṣiṇāyana: the Sun's southern progression, as tracked from the summer to the winter solstice.

Daśamī: the tenth Tithi.

Dasarā: see Vijaya Daśamī.

Devī: a name of the Goddess. See Para Śaktī

Dhaniṣṭhā: the twenty third Nakṣatra.

Dvādaśī: the twelfth Tithi.

Dvitīyā: the second Tithi.

Earth Hand: the qualities of solidity, heaviness, hardness, cold, and rigidity express in the structure and details of the hand. Earth hands have palms that are mostly square looking, short fingers, rough skin, wide, deep lines and arch fingerprints.

Eclipse: an event which occurs when an astronomical object is temporarily obscured, either by passing into the shadow of another body or by having another body pass between it and the viewer.

Ecliptic: the apparent path of the Sun. the great circle formed by the intersection of the plane of the earth's orbit with the celestial sphere; the apparent annual path of the Sun in the heavens, along which are located the 12 houses and signs of the zodiac. Aka Sūrya Marga

Ekādaśī: the eleventh Tithi.

Fire Hand: a rectangular palm with short in relation to the palm and the texture of the skin is slightly rough to the touch. The lines are strong, clear, usually reddish and tend to cross each other at odd angles creating triangles and squares and other geometric shapes. The fingerprint most associated with fire hands is the whorl.

Gaṇeśa Caturthī: is on September 8th. The culmination of a ten-day festival where Lord Ganeśa is worshipped.

Graha: 'seizer'; this word is often translated as 'planet,' but in a broader sense, means 'influencer.' Not all the grahas are physical planets. For example, the Sun is a star, and the Moon is a satellite of the earth, but they are still considered grahas.

Guru Pūrṇimā: is on July 22nd. Full-Moon holiday honoring the Guru.

Hanumān Jayantī: is on April 25th. Birthday celebration of Hanumān, the great devotee of Lord Rāma.

Hasta: the thirteenth Nakṣatra.

Hasta Sāmudrika Śāstra: also known as 'Hasta,' is the Vedic science of hand analysis, or palmistry.

Head Line: one of the primary lines in the human hand, found on every hand with no exception. It is the second horizontal line at the top of the palm. It begins on the thumb side of the hand and travels across the palm towards the little finger side. This line gives information about how a person measures their world and how they make sense of their environment.

Heart Line: the third-most significant line on the hand, following the life and head lines. It is the uppermost horizontal line on the palm, starting below the little finger and running towards the index finger. The heart line describes our emotional tendencies, the way we love, and the health of our heart as an organ.

Holī: celebrated on March 26th. Traditionally, an agriculture festival celebrating the season of Spring. 'Festival of Colors.'

Homa: Vedic rituals wherein oblations are offered into a sacred fire.

Hybrid Eclipse: under rare circumstances, a total eclipse can change to an annular eclipse or vice versa along different sections of the eclipse path, due to the curvature of the Earth.

Janma tāra: 'star of the birth'; refers to the Nakṣatra of the natal Moon at the time of birth, also called the birth star.

Japa: the repetition of a prayer, mantra or sacred formula as a vehicle for deepening one's spiritual experience. Śrī Kṛṣṇa says in the Bhagavād Gītā, "*Of the best amongst sacrifices, know me to be* japa."

Jyeṣṭhā: the eighteenth Nakṣatra.

Jyotiṣa: the ancient art and science of astrology from India. A Vedāṇga.

Kālāmṛta: 'the nectar of time.'

Karaṇa: one of the five limbs of the Pañcāṅga. Half of a Tithi.

Karma Yoga: action performed without the thirst of the results of action; also, Vaidika Karma.

Kārttika Pūrṇimā: occurs on November 16th. The Full Moon Day of the month of Kārttika.

Ketu: the south node of the Moon; the point where the Moon's path intercepts the path of the Sun in its southward motion.

Kṛṣṇa Janmāṣṭamī: is on August 28th. The birthday celebration of Lord Kṛṣṇa. The Pūja is typically performed in the evening, culminating at midnight.

Kṛṣṇa Pakṣa: the waning phase of the Moon. See Pakṣa.

Kṛttikā: the third Nakṣatra.

Krura: "cruel".

Lagna: 'to tie down'; for a natal chart, it is determined by the sign rising on the eastern horizon for a given time and place. the ascendant or rising sign.

Life Line: the principle line on the hand. Its origin is at the edge of the palm in the area between the thumb and the base of the index finger, and it curves down and around towards the wrist forming an arc around the base of the thumb. The life line provides information about the amount of life force available to us and how our life force expresses as physical strength, energy level, vitality, and recuperative ability.

Loop fingerprints: Loops flow in and out of the top part of the digit from one side and never turn into a whorl or closed shape. A person whose fingerprints are mainly loops tends to be easy-going and fit in well with others.

Lunar eclipse: can only happen during a full moon, when the Earth is between the Sun and Moon and the Earth's shadow obscures the light of the Moon.

Maghā: the tenth Nakṣatra.

Mahā Śiva Rātri: celebrated on March 9th. The great night of Śiva where an all night vigil is held in worship of the Lord.

Mahātmā: "Great Soul", one who has performed numerable deeds for the benefit of others.

Makara Saṅkrānti: on January 14th. Celebrates the Sun's entrance into the Rāśi (sign) of Capricorn.

Mālā: a rosary.

Mātṛ Rekhā: 'Rekhā' means 'line', 'Mātṛ' means 'the measurer'. See: Head Line.

Māyā: the power by which consciousness appears as the world of names and forms.

Mṛgaśīrṣa: the fifth Nakṣatra.

Muhūrta: electional astrology.

Muhūrta Cintāmaṇī: one of the traditional text books of Vedic Astrology.

Mūla: the nineteenth Nakṣatra.

Nakṣatra: one of the five limbs of the Pañcāṅga; the 27 Stars.

Namaste: a greeting, literally, "The divine in me honors the divine within you."

Navamī: the ninth Tithi.

Nirayaṇa Cakra: 'the wheel without movement'; the sidereal zodiac.

Nirguṇa: "without form", when the Supreme remains in an unmanifest state.

Oṇam: is on August 19th. A celebration in honor of the famous King Mahābali of Cera Nadu (Kerala).

Pakṣa: 'portion'; refers to the two phases of the Moon. Kṛṣṇa Pakṣa, the dark fortnight of the Moon, and Śukla Pakṣa, the bright fortnight of the Moon. Fifteen days each.

Pañcāṅga: a Vedic almanac, which contains five limbs of time, namely: Vāra, Tithi, Nakṣatra, Karaṇa, Yoga.

Pañcamī: the fifth Tithi.

Para Śaktī: the divine force that animates the Formless Oneness; an epithet of the Goddess.

Partial lunar eclipse: occurs when only a portion of the Moon enters the umbra.

Partial solar eclipses: occurs when the Moon's faint outer shadow, the Penumbra, blocks a portion of the Sun's light from a specific area on Earth.

Penumbral eclipse: occurs when the Moon passes through the Earth's penumbra. A penumbral eclipse is nearly impossible to see as the surface of the Moon is only slightly darkened

Pitṛ Pakṣa: goes from September 19th to October 4th. The fortnight of devotion to our ancestors. Pitṛ Pakṣa ends on Āmāvsyā, which is considered the most important day in the year for performing rites to our ancestors.

Prātipadā: the first Tithi.

Punarvasu: the seventh Nakṣatra.

Puṇya Kāla: 'Times of accruing merit', the best times for pursuing spiritual practice.

Pūrṇimā: the fifteenth Tithi. The full Moon.

Pūrvāṣāḍhā: the twentieth Nakṣatra.

Pūrva Bhādrapadā: the twenty-fifth Nakṣatra.

Pūrva Phalgunī: the eleventh Nakṣatra.

Puṣyā: the eighth Nakṣatra.

Rāhu: the north node of the Moon. The point where the Moon's path intercepts the path of the Sun in its northward motion.

Rāhu Kālam: an inauspicious time to begin endeavors, calculated based on the duration of the day from Sunrise to Sunset.

Rāśi: 'a heap'; the 12 signs of the zodiac.

Revatī: the twenty-seventh Nakṣatra.

Rohinī: the fourth Nakṣatra.

Ṛṣi: the sages of yore, many of whom retained a status even higher than the Gods.

Saguṇa: “with form”, referring to the Supreme when He/She takes on a form like Dakṣiṇāmūrti.

Samādhi: generally, a blissful state of the mind’s absorption in God.

Sampradāya: a lineage; sacred tradition.

Sanātana: ancient, primeval, universal.

Sanātana Dharma: original name for *Hinduism;* the Eternal Way of Righteousness.

Śaṅkarācārya: a towering intellectual who was born in 877 AD and is considered to have single handedly brought about a reformation of spiritual thought in India; *aka* Śrī Śaṅkara.

Saṅkrānti: ‘the movement of an object across a boundary.’ When a planet transits into a new Sign or Nakṣatra, especially the Sun’s transit.

Saptamī: the seventh Tithi.

Sarasvatī Pūjā: on February 14th. Festival of the Goddess Sarasvatī. Celebrated on the fifth lunar day of the month of Māgha. Also known as Vasant Pañcamī, the beginning of spring.

Saros: a period of 223 synodic months that can be used to predict eclipses of the Sun and Moon.

Sāyana cakra: ‘the moving wheel’; the tropical zodiac, which aligns to the seasons through solstices.

Śārad Navarātrī: begins on October 5th. The nine nights of the Goddess. It signals the beginning of winter and celebrates the slaying of Mahiśāsura by the goddess Dūrgā. Culminates with Vijaya Daśamī. Worship Durgā is performed the first three days of the festival, Lakṣmī the second three days and Sarasvatī during the last three days of the festival.

Ṣaṣṭhī: the sixth Tithi.

Śatabhīṣā: the twenty-fourth Nakṣatra.

Śiva: the Lord of dissolving creation; Śiva is the śānta (peaceful) form of Lord Rudra.

Solar eclipse: can only occur during a new Moon when the Sun's light becomes obstructed by the Moon passing in front of it, as observed from Earth.

Śravaṇa: the twenty-second Nakṣatra.

Śukla Pakṣa: the waxing phase of the Moon. See Pakṣa.

Śruti: the Vedas; literally, 'that which is heard.'

Stotra: a Sanskrit work, both poetic and often spiritual by nature.

Sūrya: the Sun.

Sūrya Siddhānta: the king of all traditional text books on astronomical calculation in India, supplying astronomical formulas as revealed by the Sun God himself.

Svāti: the fifteenth Nakṣatra.

Tāra Bala: 'strength of the star'; refers to the relationship between Janma Tāra and the star of the day.

Tithi: one of the five limbs of the Pañcāṅga; the 30 lunar days from one new Moon to the next new Moon.

Titikṣā: 'accommodation'. The ability to accept the circumstances that life presents.

Total lunar eclipse: occurs when the Moon is completely swallowed by the Earths umbra. In a full lunar eclipse, the Moon passes through all the stages – Penumbral, Partial and Full.

Total solar eclipse: occurs when the Earth falls into the dark center or the umbra portion of the Moon's shadow and therefore the disk of the Sun is fully obscured by the Moon.

Trayodaśī: the thirteenth Tithi.

Tṛtīyā: the third Tithi.

Uttara Aṣāḍhā: the twenty-first Nakṣatra.

Uttarāyaṇa: the Sun's northern progression as tracked from the winter to the summer solstice.

Uttara Bhādrapadā: the twenty-sixth Nakṣatra.

Uttara Phalgunī: the twelfth Nakṣatra.

Vaikuṇṭha: the world and dwelling place of Lord Viṣṇu and Goddess Lakṣmī.

Vāra: one of the five limbs of the Pañcāṅga; a weekday.

Vārāhamihīra: great astronomer and astrologer. He is considered to be one of the nine jewels of the court of King Vikramāditya.

Vijaya Daśamī: is on October 13th. The final day of Navarātrī. Also,known as Dasarā, where in some places an effigy of Rāvaṇa is burnt to celebrate Rāma's victory over Rāvaṇa. One of the four most auspicious days of the year.

Viśākhā: the sixteenth Nakṣatra.

Viṣṇu: the God responsible for the cosmic function of sustaining creation.

Viṣu (or Meṣa Saṅkrānti): is on April 14th. The Sun's movement into the Rāśi (Sign) of Aries. The solar New Year,.

Yoga: one of the five limbs of the Pañcāṅga. A particular relationship of the Sun and Moon.

Water hands: Narrow, rectangular palms with the longest fingers of all the hand types, the fingers are often delicate and very flexible. The water hand is the most refined of all the hand types. The ... palm of the water type is covered with a great number of fine lines, with the principal lines standing out from the rest. The lines are usually thin, forming a shallow, web-like, tangled mass. The fingerprint pattern most associated with the water hand is the loop.

Whorl Fingerprint : a pattern of concentric circles that typically is seen on a fire hand. Attributes include; individuality, uniqueness and intensity.

CONTRIBUTORS

Śrī Pūrṇa has always had a deep love for astrology. She began studying Vedic Astrology, palmistry, Vāstu and Sanskrit with her beloved teacher Hart de Fouw in 2001. Along with her husband Michael, she is a resident astrologer for the M.A. Math. When not traveling with Amma, she enjoys teaching Jyotiṣa in the form of classes as well as private tutorings. She offers readings, palmistry and Vāstu consults worldwide.

Sripurna.jyotish@gmail.com
www.kalamrita.com

Michael Bonvino, a student of Mr. Hart de Fouw, is a practitioner of Jyotiṣa for the M.A. Math and travels with Amma offering Jyotiṣa consultations. Michael also leads annual guided temple tours to the temples of Tamiḷ Nadu.

Mbonvino108@yahoo.com
www.kalamrita.com
www.paramokshatours.com

Claudia Anfuso is a student and practitioner of Jyotiṣa (Vedic Astrology), as well as of Hindu Palmistry. In 2006 she took her first of many courses in Hasta Sāmudrika (Hindu hand analysis) with world renowned Jyotiṣa master Hart de Fouw. That course ignited a life-long passion for the human hand and its encoding of both character and destiny patterns. Claudia delights in teaching both palmistry basics and in-depth workshops on this sacred art.

Claudia@considerastrology.com
www.ConsiderAstrology.com

Kālāmṛta 2013

We would love to hear about how you use Kālāmṛta!

Let us know, along with suggestions for future editions:

Kalamrita@gmail.com

And stop by our place for a bit:

www.kalamrita.com

Help us to determine the deity for Kālāmṛta 2014! Email us a *single* suggestion of your favorite Hindu God or Goddess and if yours is the one chosen, you will automatically be entered into a raffle along with other people who had the same suggestion. The winner will receive a free Kālāmṛta 2014 & 2015. We'll choose three winners so send us your suggestions!

Notes: